yoga

for pain relief

A NEW APPROACH TO AN ANCIENT PRACTICE

LEE ALBERT, NMT

FOREWORD BY PEGGY CAPPY

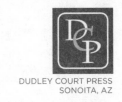

DUDLEY COURT PRESS
SONOITA, AZ

Dudley Court Press
PO Box 102
Sonoita, AZ 85637
www.DudleyCourtPress.com

Connect with Lee Albert at www.LeeAlbert.com

Cover and interior design by Dunn+Associates, www.Dunn-Design.com

ISBN: 978-1-940013-32-9
LCCN: 2017931869

Publisher's Cataloging-in-Publication Data
Albert, Lee (Lee Michael), 1951- author. | Cappy, Peggy, writer of foreword.
Yoga for pain relief: a new approach to an ancient practice
Lee Albert: Sonoita, AZ : Dudley Court Press, [2017] |
"Foreword by Peggy Cappy"—Cover. | Includes index.
ISBN: 978-1-940013-32-9 | LCCN: 2017931869
LCSH: Yoga—Therapeutic use. | Yoga—Study and teaching. | Pain—Treatment. | Analgesia. |
Meditation—Therapeutic use. | Breathing exercises—Therapeutic use.
Classification:
LCC: RM727.Y64 A43 2017 | DDC: 613.7/046—dc23

To my wife Marcia for her love, support and encouragement

To my publisher Gail for her expertise and dedication

To Peggy Cappy for her enthusiasm and dedication
to bringing this information to as many people as possible

To all my clients and students who have taught me so much

To all the amazing people on this planet who are taking responsibility for their experiences
in life and are making the commitment to do something about it

If you always do what you've always done,

you will always get what you've always got.

If you want things that you never got,

you must do things you have never done!

—Nishan Panwar

contents

foreword

You are holding in your hands an important book.

I know this from direct experience. Years ago, I returned to the U.S. after an extended meditation retreat in India. Prolonged hours of sitting in Ardha Padmasana (Half Lotus Pose) resulted in an excruciating pain in my right hip. It was so severe I thought at first I might need a hip replacement.

When I determined that my problem was muscular rather than in the joint, I knew where to go and who to see. Lee Albert. I found him at Kripalu Center for Yoga and Health where I regularly teach Yoga for the Rest of Us. Each time I am at Kripalu, I attend Lee's one-hour sampler called Live Pain-Free. It is astonishing and heart-warming to watch Lee work with volunteers from the audience. You know you are in the presence of a gifted man when you see those people leave the session pain-free. I could hardly wait for Lee to work on me.

Two minutes. That's what it took to fix my hip pain. I can still remember saying, "It's like a miracle! I simply can't believe that the pain is gone. It took only two minutes of your holding my leg in that gentle yoga stretch."

Lee's work, Integrated Positional Therapy, comes from his own personal experience and his search for relief from the severe pain he suffered as a result of a horrible car accident. Though Lee's work may at first seem unbelievable, even miraculous, due to such immediate and extraordinary results, I promise you his remedies are gentle and effective, yet powerful and rapid. And lasting. My hip no longer hurts. The pain has never returned, thanks to my learning which muscles to stretch to keep my body in neuromuscular balance.

Having known and worked with Lee Albert for many years, I am honored and delighted to introduce his newest book to you. While many books on Yoga are published each year, *Yoga for Pain Relief, A New Approach to an Ancient Practice* is destined to rock the Yoga world. Lee sheds new light on how yoga solutions can be used therapeutically to create pain-free living.

In this book Lee gives us the key to practicing Yoga safely while achieving superior results. Lee will introduce you to the five major muscle imbalances from which most of us suffer, and how to correct them with common yoga poses. Most importantly, he addresses the root cause of pain.

I encourage you to read *Yoga for Pain Relief* and put it into practice. Select the yoga postures that will most benefit your current body conditions, or those of your students if you teach Yoga. Your results will be all the evidence you need to recognize and appreciate this new approach to the ancient practice of Yoga.

Wishing you pain-free living and tremendous well-being,

Peggy Cappy

CEO of Peggy Cappy Enterprises; author of *Yoga for All of Us,*
A Modified Series of Traditional Poses for Any Age and Ability;
creator of *Yoga for the Rest of Us* video series;
popular TV host of PBS Yoga programming since 2002

preface

the book you are about to read had its origin thirty years ago. At that time I had no idea I was going to write a book, nor did I even have the desire to write one. I could not have possibly foreseen the events that would bring me to this place in my life. I am now compelled to share the knowledge I have gained since that day when my life was propelled in a new direction. This story will be familiar to readers of my first book, *Live Pain-free without Drugs or Surgery.*

I will always remember that day. The weather was beautiful and sunny, and I was driving peacefully along the road in the gorgeous countryside of Quebec, Canada. I gently pressed the brakes and came to a stop at a stop sign. In my rearview mirror, I saw a car traveling at a high speed quickly closing in on me. Before I could react, three thousand pounds of glass and steel moving at fifty to sixty miles an hour slammed into my car.

Looking back on that moment, I consider myself lucky. I escaped from this horrific accident with no noticeable injuries. My car was not as fortunate: it was a mangled mess. I was taken to a local hospital to be examined by a doctor. My vital signs were all normal, and to tell you the truth, I felt fine. The doctor assured me that everything was all right but that I should check in with my doctor when I got home.

My story could have ended there, but it was unfortunately only beginning. Three weeks after the accident, I developed a terrible headache. This pain was different from the occasional headaches I would sometimes experience. I would later learn that what I was experiencing was a migraine. Little did I know that I would have these headaches quite often for the next three years.

The doctor prescribed pain relievers. Unfortunately, they did little to help and often made me nauseous. I did not wish to live my life with this pain. The doctors had few other suggestions that would help me. I knew that if I were going to get better, I would have to find the answers to these headaches on my own.

The doctors identified the cause of my migraines as muscular tension in my neck, or severe whiplash as it is more commonly called. Thus, I began my search to learn everything I could about the musculoskeletal system. I wanted to know how tight muscles cause pain and what therapies were the most effective at relieving pain.

I became a massage therapist and eventually a neuromuscular therapist. I also received training in orthopedic massage and myofascial release. I was learning a great deal about the body as I diligently studied musculoskeletal anatomy. But though I received many forms of bodywork twice a week, still my headaches persisted.

The technique that finally relieved me of my headaches was positional therapy, which is sometimes called strain/counterstrain therapy. This gentle but effective therapy takes strain off muscles and resets them to normal resting length, thus reducing pain and bringing the muscles back into balance. I felt I'd experienced a miracle when my headaches finally went away after all those years. I was curious to know why positional therapy worked when other techniques did not. What was the "secret" that gave me this blessed relief? That answer was still awaiting me.

In furthering my studies about the body, I studied yoga. I underwent teacher's training and eventually became a yoga teacher. I liked the way my body felt when I practiced. Yoga also opened my eyes to the benefits of pranayama (breathing) and meditation as powerful tools for pain relief and well-being.

Still, something was missing. In general, I felt relaxed and energized after my yoga practice. However, sometimes certain yoga postures did not feel so good and even verged on painful. I did not like that feeling, but I thought at the time that the pain was simply showing me where my restrictions were and that I needed to work harder to break through those barriers. So I stretched deeper and longer. In hindsight, my thinking was faulty.

Concurrently, as a neuromuscular therapist, I noticed I was treating more and more people who were injured while practicing yoga. At first I thought the reason was because the yogis and yoginis were a little too exuberant in their practice. Were they stretching too deeply? My other thought was that maybe participants were not warming up their muscles well enough before practicing, or they were doing advanced poses they were not ready for.

However, my theories didn't add up. I know from experience that most yoga practitioners are in touch with their bodies, and they are careful and thoughtful about their practice. How could it be that I was treating an increasing number of yoga injuries?

Then one day, I found the missing link, and the "secret" was suddenly evident. I combined my knowledge of yoga with the knowledge I'd gained from my bodywork studies, especially in positional therapy. The answer was staring me in the face for quite a while, but I hadn't been able to see it. Surprisingly, you can find information about it on the Internet. Some physical therapists and neuromuscular therapists are familiar with this simple but fundamental concept. I further developed this concept into a protocol (Integrated Positional Therapy) that I now use in my yoga teaching and body work practice to achieve a greater degree of pain relief and well-being with longer-lasting results.

Although the concept I've learned is not currently well known by yoga practitioners, I believe it is the key to practicing yoga safely and achieving superior results. Once you learn about this crucial principle, it will catapult your yoga practice to a whole new level. When the yoga world starts adopting this not-so-well-kept secret, yoga could become the therapy that people seek out first when they have musculoskeletal pain. By using the principles in your yoga practice that I am going to teach you, you will be addressing the root cause of your pain.

I am eager to share with you the wisdom I have learned on my journey to wholeness. I want you to know that you, too, can achieve a pain-free body and have a sense of well-being by applying the information in this book to your yoga practice both on and off the yoga mat. I am going to give you the tools to not only reduce or eliminate the pain in your life but to show you how to be more fully alive. These tools will help you to achieve your true potential—which is nothing short of greatness!

January 25, 2017
Pittsfield, Massachusetts

introduction

how to use this book

do you or your yoga students struggle with tight hamstrings, sore knees, back pain, or hips that won't open? Is your stress making you sick? Do you feel anxious and find it difficult to relax and be calm? Is there an effective way to deal with these conditions through yoga? There sure is.

The focus of this book is yoga practice for well-being and pain relief using modern yoga. The ancient yogis believed that a regular yoga practice could help with all aspects of one's being. Since our life-styles today are quite different from that of the ancient yogis, we will benefit by culling the traditional yoga practices that will most benefit our needs in the twenty-first century. The information I present is suitable for those new to yoga and for those who have been practicing for many years, both students and teachers. This material is for those who want to be able to achieve even better results from their yoga practice and for those who are struggling with certain poses and conditions. It is suitable for all body types.

In the following chapters we will discuss the powerful benefits of asana (stretching), pran-ayama (breathing) and meditation, especially as they apply to neuromuscular conditions and the general health of the body, mind, and spirit. These tools of the ancient yogis are making resurgence in our modern world as science is confirming their many benefits.

In the final analysis, most pain is foundational, resulting from imbalances in the musculo-skeletal system. We are in pain because we are misaligned, or "crooked." We have poor posture as a result. Even if you think you have good posture, you probably don't, as misalignments are often not obvious to the untrained eye. The following chapters will teach you how to identify the most common misalignments and to develop a quick and simple approach to better posture and muscle balance.

By incorporating this information into your practice, you will be able to more precisely choose the poses best suited for your current body conditions. Yoga should not be about performing poses but rather selecting the poses that will most benefit your current body conditions. Not all yoga postures are suitable for all individuals. Depending on your postural imbalances, you might need to avoid certain poses until the body is back in balance. The information I am presenting will help identify these imbalances, explain how current poses you are practicing might be causing or contributing to pain, and show you how to develop a yoga practice that can achieve the right balance for you. The result will be less pain and more vitality in your life.

Western medicine has few interventions for the musculoskeletal pain and stress often caused by our modern lifestyles. Typically, doctors prescribe painkillers, muscle relaxers, and antianxiety drugs. These can often bring some relief, but they are only treating the symptoms rather than the root problem.

Selecting the correct asanas (poses) for your particular musculoskeletal condition requires some knowledge of anatomy and muscle imbalances. Knowing how to deal with the stress and anxiety in our daily lives requires some knowledge of the mind and body. These yoga solutions will help you alleviate the root causes of your conditions.

I have trained thousands of people in my workshops, including MDs, physical therapists, chiropractors, massage therapists, and lay people. They have all learned how easy it is to reduce or eliminate pain. They have learned how to achieve a greater sense of well-being when following my protocols.

In the following pages, I want to take you on a journey. You will discover:

• the roots of yoga, and how traditional yoga differs from what we practice today

• the miraculous mechanics of your musculoskeletal system

• the cause of most aches and pains

• how to reduce pain and achieve better results from your practice

• how to select the correct asanas for you and your students' conditions

• why people get hurt practicing yoga and how to avoid injury

• how to stretch

• specific yoga flows for pain relief

• guidelines for achieving superior results

• the many benefits of pranayama and meditation

• how to reduce or eliminate stress and anxiety

• how to integrate yoga into your everyday life

• and much more.

Please read each chapter in the order I present them. Each one builds on the last to give you the knowledge you need to take your practice to the next level so you can eliminate many painful conditions.

Let's get started!

CHAPTER 1

a balanced body is a pain-free body

"Yoga is the study of balance, and balance is the aim of all living creatures: it is our home."
—**Rolf Gates**

at least one hundred million Americans suffer from chronic pain. Chronic pain is defined as pain lasting longer than six months. That number goes much higher when we add the statistics for acute pain. Chronic and acute pain can range from mild to moderate to excruciating. Dealing with pain costs society over $600 billion dollars each and every year. This is a significant public health problem.

As a neuromuscular therapist, I have observed that the four most common complaints from my clients are back pain, neck pain, headaches, and knee pain. In fact, I will bet that many of you reading this book have suffered with some of these conditions or know someone who has. Chronic and acute pain will likely affect most people at some time in their lives.

Interestingly, back in the 1950s when I was growing up, low back pain was one of the most common reasons that compelled a person to seek medical help. Today in 2017, low back pain is still one of the most common reasons a person will seek medical attention. How can it be that in a country with such an advanced medical system that low back pain is still so persistent?

The answer is that usually when a doctor or therapist treats low back pain, they are treating symptoms, not the cause. Of course, treating the symptoms to achieve relief is well and good, but in the long term treating the cause of the low back pain will yield longer-term relief.

A great deal of research presents evidence that the root cause of many neuromuscular pain patterns is due to biomechanical malalignments caused by muscle imbalances. Therapists often refer to this as the muscles being locked long or locked short.

When you visit your doctor, you could be diagnosed with any one of hundreds of conditions. In our Western model of medicine, standard treatment for conditions like sciatica, plantar fasciitis, carpal tunnel, tennis elbow, low back pain, most headaches, and herniated discs involves treating the symptoms, typically with a painkiller or an anti-inflammatory drug. Seldom does Western medicine treat the cause.

I am now going to reveal to you the "secret" I became aware of that finally relieved my headaches after the car accident. I use this knowledge almost daily to help people reduce or eliminate their neuro-muscular pain. The secret is correcting muscle imbalances. In my experience, these imbalances can account for 80% of the pain a person will experience in their lifetime! Correcting muscle imbalances will give you better posture, more energy, and reduce or eliminate many painful conditions.

Muscle imbalances are often the cause of many painful conditions you will experience in your life, including:

- Tension-type headaches and migraines
- Temporomandibular joint disorder (TMJD)
- Cervical muscle strain (neck pain)
- Thoracic outlet syndrome (TOS)
- Epicondylitis, lateral or medial (tennis or golfer's elbow)
- Carpal tunnel syndrome (CTS)
- Lumbar muscle strain (low back pain)
- Piriformis syndrome (sciatica)
- Medial meniscus injury (knee pain)
- Plantar fasciitis (heel spur)
- Fibromyalgia
- Disc abnormalities
- Nerve compressions
- Fascial restrictions
- Poor posture
- Knee and hip replacements
- Reduced flow in the energetic body (prana)
- . . . and many more painful conditions.

what is a muscle imbalance?

A muscle imbalance occurs when muscles become either too long or too short. Muscles that are too short or long will cause the muscular system to become painful and possibly even inflamed.

Optimal functioning of the musculoskeletal system requires that muscles be in balance in regard to strength and length. If muscles do not possess this balance, they become painful, and the joint where these imbalances occur will become compromised. This often manifests as pain in that joint and/or limited range of motion.

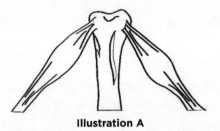

Illustration A

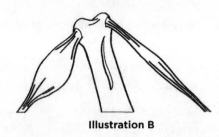

Illustration B

Illustration A demonstrates what muscles in balance look like. They are equal length and strength. **Illustration B** demonstrates what a muscle imbalance looks like. Notice that the muscle on the left is short and contracted. (This muscle is then considered strong.) The muscle on the right is too long and overstretched. (This muscle is then considered weak.) These small imbalances will cause the bigger imbalances we see in the next diagram.

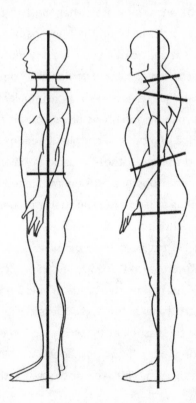

The figure on the left is what a balanced body looks like. The figure on the right has numerous muscle imbalances. Most people exhibit at least some of these imbalances and are not even aware that they have muscle imbalances. Another way to think about imbalances is to look at your posture. If you have poor posture, you have muscle imbalances like the figure on the right. If your muscles are in balance, you have good posture like the figure on the left. To be concise, a muscle imbalance is when some muscles are too short and tight, and some muscles are too long and tight.

When muscles become too short, they will feel tight and will often become achy or painful. Now, pay close attention to this next statement. **When muscles become too long, they also will**

feel tight and will often become achy or painful. At first this doesn't seem to make much sense. Let's take a closer look.

Imagine a rubber band. Imagine that you are now pulling two ends of the rubber band farther apart. This stretching of the rubber band is making it longer and tighter, is it not?

Let's experience this in our bodies. A common muscle imbalance in our culture is that many people have their shoulders rounded forward. This is due to improperly sitting in a chair. Try this now. Round your shoulders forward by contracting your chest muscles. Touch the chest muscles and they will feel tight, as you would expect. Now touch the upper back muscles between your shoulder blades. You will notice they also feel tight. As a matter of fact, they feel much tighter than the short muscles in most people. Muscles that are too long and tight often feel substantially tighter than muscles that are too short and tight.

When muscles are out of balance, they are either too short and tight or too long and tight. This is the knowledge we need in order to bring the body back into balance.

You are probably wondering at this point if you have any muscle imbalances. The answer is yes, you do. Almost everyone has muscle imbalances. If you sit at a computer, drive a car or watch TV for more than an hour a day, you most likely have some muscle imbalances. Poor posture is a telltale sign. If the imbalances are small, you probably don't have any symptoms. If the imbalances are significant, you will have pain and limited range of motion in certain directions.

Since muscles are attached to bones, these muscle imbalances pull the bones out of alignment, and that's what gives you poor posture. Muscle imbalances also put abnormal strain on the tendons and ligaments. A tendon is a band of tissue that attaches a muscle to a bone. A ligament is a band of tissue that attaches a bone to another bone.

Misalignment of the skeletal structure caused by muscle imbalances can cause compressions of the nerves, discs, and other structures in the body. It can also cause the fascia to be twisted and restricted. Fascia is a band of fibrous connective tissue enveloping, separating, or binding together muscles, organs, and other soft structures of the body. These twists, compressions, and tight muscles ultimately lead to less oxygen in the tissues at those areas. The medical term for this is ischemia, which means that the blood getting to the tissues is inadequate. Since blood is the carrier of oxygen, the tissue is not getting enough oxygen. **This lack of oxygen is the source of a lot of pain.**

what causes most muscle imbalances?

We commonly acquire muscle imbalances in three ways: by overusing certain muscles, keeping muscles in an unbalanced position, and by overstretching.

By using one muscle more intensely and frequently than its opposing muscle, it will become too short, thus pulling the opposing muscle too long. A common example is when people ride bicycles. When riding a bike, the quadriceps muscle group on the front of the upper thigh is used to push the pedals. The hamstrings on the back of the upper thigh are not used nearly as much when riding a bike. This exercise will make the quadriceps shorter and stronger, thus pulling the hamstrings on the back of the upper thigh into a longer and weaker condition. These overstretched, too long hamstrings will feel tight. Because they feel tight, most people think they have short hamstrings, which is not the case at all.

Here is a key concept to remember: Muscles that are too long usually feel much tighter than muscles that are too short. Until you can identify the muscle as too short and tight or too long and tight, you will not know what pose to select to correct the imbalance.

Another way we commonly acquire muscle imbalances is by keeping the muscles in an imbalanced condition for long periods of time. The most common example is sitting in a chair. When sitting in a chair, the quadriceps muscles go into a shortened and strong position that, of course, pulls the hamstring muscles into a long and weak position. Given that most people sit at least several hours a day (computer, driving, etc.), we have now trained the hamstrings and quadriceps to be out of balance.

Stretching the same muscles over and over again and ignoring others can develop muscle imbalances. This often happens when a yoga practitioner or athlete stretches the same muscles and ignores others at every practice. Stretching muscles that are already too long also will make your muscle imbalances more pronounced. Stretching muscles that are too long is a common but easy mistake when practicing yoga because the muscle does feel tight, and stretching it does make it feel looser.

Let's look at a common example. Many people present with a forward (anterior) tilt to their pelvis due to short, tight hip flexors (rectus femoris and psoas). This tilt will often lead to low back pain, an exaggerated lumbar curve, and a feeling of tight hamstrings. Since muscles work in pairs, if the hip flexors are too short, the hamstrings (one of the hip extensors) must be too long. So, of course, most people believe you should stretch the hamstrings. The stretching will make it feel better and looser, but ultimately you are increasing the imbalance by making the hamstrings even longer.

Kyle Stull, in his enlightening article, explains the mechanism by which this occurs:

> An example of this is the person with an anterior pelvic tilt (excessive arch in the low back). As the pelvis tilts forward, the hamstrings are lengthened. Over time, these muscles begin to feel "tight." In most cases, the individual will feel the need to stretch the hamstrings. As the hamstrings are stretched, the GTO (Golgi tendon organ) will inhibit the muscle spindles (autogenic inhibition) and the hamstrings will begin to feel as though they have relaxed. Yet this altered position of the pelvis causes a lengthened resting position of the muscle, and as soon as the GTO is no longer excited the muscle spindle will begin to signal for the CNS to contract, leading to reoccurring tightness.
>
> —http://blog.nasm.org/cex/overactive-versus-underactive-muscles-mean/#sthash.s00sZXpR.dpuf

What Kyle Stull is saying is that even though the hamstrings feel tight, they are not short, and stretching them will not bring them back into balance. Many people that I treat in my private practice have tight hamstrings. Most of them believe that they should be stretching the hamstrings. Seldom have I ever treated someone with a short hamstring. They are tight, but they are overstretched tight. The correct course of action is to make them shorter, which will help them to relax into the balanced position.

How to identify Muscel imBalances?.

myth

My tight hamstrings are too short, so stretching them is the solution.

fact

Short hamstrings are rare. Tight hamstrings are common, but they are not usually short; they are too long and tight.

Identify your current muscle imbalances first, then select the proper pose or exercise that will bring the muscles and bones into balance.

Muscle imbalances can either be developed or exacerbated by doing the wrong yoga pose, Pilates exercise, or strength training exercise for your current musculoskeletal condition. When practicing yoga, Pilates, or working out in the gym, you will achieve superior results by first identifying your muscle imbalances. Failure to do so will eventually result in some painful condition in the body. It is not adequate to identify a muscle as tight. If you do not know if it is short tight or too long tight, you simply do not know what action to take, i.e. what pose or exercise to practice to correct this imbalance.

fun fact The ancient Chinese recognized this imbalance between the quadriceps and hamstrings. They knew that people who walk upright did not use their hamstrings nearly as much as their quads. Their solution was to walk up hills backward to strengthen the hamstrings. This practice would make the hamstrings shorter and stronger and thus bring them back into balance.

If you try this practice yourself, you will quickly see how weak your hamstrings are. I do not recommend this practice, as there are better ways to strengthen the hamstrings that we will learn about in later chapters.

focus on these five major imbalances

Recognizing muscle imbalances is imperative so you can select the correct pose that will help to bring the body into balance and out of pain. This endeavor is not nearly as difficult as one might expect. Since most people perform similar activities during their lives, most people present with similar muscle imbalances with variations on a theme.

The easiest way to identify muscle imbalances is to remember that in the beginning most people will present with muscles on the anterior (front side) of their body too short and muscles on the posterior (back side) too long except for the calves, which are typically too short. In my experience, the primary cause of this pattern is a lifetime of sitting in chairs.

Start looking at people and observing their posture. You will soon see that most people present exactly like I am telling you—too short in the front and too long in the back. Their heads are forward, chest collapsed, and the body bent forward at the waist.

The body can have many imbalances, but following are the five major imbalances. Once corrected, most of the smaller imbalances will fall into place. When you know what to look for, it is pretty obvious.

What to look for	Muscle imbalance 1	Symptoms
Pelvis higher on one side	Short quadratus lumborum	Low back pain
One leg shorter than the other		Knee pain
		Sacroiliac pain
		Disc issues
		Scoliosis

What to look for	Muscle imbalance 2	Symptoms
Pelvis rotated	Short piriformis	Low back pain
Feet & legs rotated laterally	Short hip abductors	Hip pain
	Long hip adductors	Knee pain
		Groin pain
		Sacroiliac pain
		Disc pain

What to look for	Muscle imbalance 3	Symptoms
Pelvis tilted forward	Short quads	Hamstring pain or tightness
Exaggerated lumbar curve	Short psoas	Knee pain
	Long hamstrings	Sacroiliac pain
		Low back pain
		Disc pain

What to look for	Muscle imbalance 4	Symptoms
Head forward/ shoulders forward	Short neck flexors	Neck pain
	Long neck extensors	Headaches
	Short pectorals	TMJ
	Long rhomboids	Sunken chest
		Upper back pain

What to look for	Muscle imbalance 5	Symptoms
Head tilted to side/elevated shoulder	Short scalene	Neck pain
	Short levator scapula	Chest pain
		Arm pain
		Hand pain
		Shoulder pain

Yoga can correct these muscle imbalances in a relatively short time once you learn how to choose the correct stretches for your symptoms. In chapter 2 we will learn about the brilliant mechanics of the human machine. We will learn the language of anatomy. This will be helpful in understanding muscle imbalances and the root causes of most painful neuromuscular conditions. This information will be useful in selecting the correct pose for your current imbalances.

Key Points

- **Muscle imbalances** account for 80% of the pain you will experience in your life.

- **Poor posture** is a telltale sign of muscle imbalances.

- **Muscle imbalances** are caused by overusing certain muscles and underusing others.

- **Muscles that are too long** usually feel much tighter than muscles that are too short. Until you can identify the muscle as too short and tight or too long and tight, you will not know what pose to select to correct the imbalance.

- **Muscle imbalances** can either be developed or exacerbated by doing the wrong yoga pose, Pilates exercise, or strength training exercise for your current musculo-skeletal condition.

- **In general, muscles on the backside of the body are too long,** except for the calves. Muscles on the front side of the body are too short.

- **Stretching muscles** that are already too long is a common mistake in yoga class.

- **There are five major muscle imbalances** you need to identify.

- **Yoga can correct these muscle imbalances** in a relatively short time once you learn how to choose the correct poses for your symptoms.

- **Correcting muscle imbalances** will give you better posture, more energy, and reduce or eliminate many painful conditions.

a quick (not too technical) course in anatomy

"Our own physical body possesses a wisdom which we who inhabit the body lack. We give it orders which make no sense."
—Henry Miller

anatomy class. Those two words often cause a great deal of anxiety. One of my students summed it up nicely: "All those Latin words that nobody can pronounce, hundreds of muscles, hundreds of bones, and miles of nerves. Even if I learn all the names, which seems rather daunting, how will I ever figure out how they all work together?" Good question!

Anatomy is truly a lifelong study that is fascinating and enlightening. I encourage everyone to study as much as they can about their own human machine. However, I know most people are completely overwhelmed with just thinking about all that anatomy and probably will not delve too deeply into the subject.

In this book, I am going to teach you the bare bone basics that will be required to take your practice to the next level and bring the body into balance. You will see the topic is far from overwhelming, and most people are pleasantly surprised to see how easy it is. I also believe that it would have been to our benefit to learn this knowledge of the body in grade school. You will see in later chapters how this pertains to your yoga practice, and it will all come together for you.

A basic understanding of some of the systems in the body will be helpful in our study of asana—in particular the skeletal, fascial, nervous, and muscular systems.

the skeletal system

The human body has 206 bones. The skeletal system performs vital functions—support, protection, blood cell production, calcium storage, and endocrine regulation—that enable us to move through our daily lives.

A typical bone has a dense and tough outer layer. Next is a layer of spongy bone, which is lighter and slightly flexible. In the middle of some bones is jelly-like bone marrow, where new cells are constantly making new blood. Bones protect many of the vital organs.

The place where two bones meet is called a joint. Ligaments are bands of tissue that connect these bones. Proper alignment of these bones is essential for optimal functioning.

fun fact : *Teeth are considered part of the skeletal system but are not counted as bones.*

the fascial system

This greatly misunderstood system is talked about more and more as many people are discovering its vital role in the body. The easiest way to think about fascia is like a continuous sheath that runs from head to toe without interruption, the "glue" that holds everything together. Often described as looking and reacting much like a spider web, it is the means by which each part of the body is connected to every other part. Another name for fascia is connective tissue. Fascia interpenetrates other soft tissue in the body. You cannot stretch muscle without stretching fascia, and vice versa.

fun fact : *The fascia has ten times more sensory nerve endings than our muscles.*

the nervous system

The nervous system is like the electrical wiring in your house or car. Its basic function is to send signals from one part of the body to others. The central nervous system is connected to every part of the body by forty-three pairs of nerves. Twelve pairs run to and from the brain, with thirty-one pairs branching out from the spinal cord. Nerves often become compressed and irritated due to an imbalance in the muscular system.

fun fact : *Our bodies have nearly forty-five miles of nerves running through them.*

the muscular system

Muscles in the body are divided into three types: smooth, cardiac, and skeletal.

Smooth muscles are the involuntary muscles controlled by the autonomic nervous system. They help the body do its everyday jobs that keep it running smoothly. They are often found on the inside of internal organs. For example, these muscles automatically contract the wall of your intestine to move food through it or contract your bladder to eliminate urine.

Cardiac muscle refers to the heart tissue. These muscles are also involuntary and help move the blood throughout the body. Cardiac muscle contracts to move the blood out of the heart and relaxes to fill it with blood again.

Over six hundred skeletal muscles are attached to bones by way of connective tissue called tendons. Skeletal muscles and tendons work together to move bones in relation to each other. A skeletal muscle produces movement, stabilizes joints, and maintains posture. Those close to the skin are called superficial muscles, and those closest to the inside of the body are called the deep muscles. These skeletal muscles are under our voluntary control. They are typically paired together in sets that work in conjunction with one another. They come in various sizes and perform many different functions. These are the muscles we are mainly working with in our practice of yoga.

fun facts : *The smallest muscle in the human body, located in the inner ear, is called the stapedius.*

The largest muscle in the human body is the gluteus maximus, located in the buttocks.

The longest muscle in the human body is called the sartorius, located in the upper leg.

what you absolutely need to know about muscles

This book will focus on the skeletal muscular system as we explore our approach to asana practice. The other systems I talked about above (skeletal, nervous, and fascial) are impacted by the muscular system. By learning a few key concepts on how the muscular system works, we can help bring those other systems into balance as well.

muscles often work in pairs

The two parts of the pair are called the agonist and the antagonist. The agonist is the prime mover, the major muscle causing the movement. Smaller muscles called synergistic muscles often aid the agonist. When the agonist contracts (becomes shorter), its opposite muscle, the antagonist, must relax (becomes longer). These skeletal muscles produce motion by pulling on the bones in this manner. Let me give you an example.

The biceps are the muscles on the front of the upper arm. Contract your biceps muscles by bringing your hand toward your shoulder. This movement will make your biceps bulge a little. In this position the bicep muscles have become shorter due to the contraction. The muscles located on the back of the upper arm (triceps) have become longer. In this case, the biceps are the agonist and the triceps are the antagonist.

Now let's reverse the process by making the arm straight. This time you are contracting the triceps (making them shorter) and stretching your biceps (making them longer). In this case, the triceps are the agonist and the biceps are the antagonist.

An agonist muscle that is stronger than the corresponding antagonist muscle can lead to a muscular imbalance. The muscular imbalance pulls the skeletal system out of alignment and can lead to nerve impingements, disc abnormalities, and fascial restrictions.

muscles develop imbalances due to over or underuse

In our daily lives, we have all developed habits that impact our muscular system. These habits are things we usually do every day, such as our jobs, the way we sit, and what we choose for exercise or don't choose for exercise. All of our daily actions require that we use or don't use our muscles in a certain way. Some of our muscles we use frequently and some we use far less. This can lead to the muscles becoming imbalanced.

The muscles we use often will tend to get shorter, and the muscles we use less often tend to get longer. The way we sit also puts some muscles in a shorter position and some in a longer position often for extended periods of time. For example, when you are slumping in a chair, your chest muscles have become shorter, and the muscles between your shoulder blades (rhomboids) have become longer.

myth

My upper back muscles feel really tight and sore, so they must be too short.

fact

Muscles that are too long often feel tighter and are usually more painful than short muscles. Upper back muscles are usually too long.

some muscles are weak, and some are strong

We often refer to muscles as being weak or strong. What we are observing is the relationship of a muscle to its opposite. To use our chest example again, when the chest muscles are habitually contracted, pulling the head forward and rounding the shoulders, they are considered strong because they are winning the battle with the upper back muscles. The upper back muscles then are considered weak because they do not have enough strength to pull the head and shoulders back into alignment. Muscles that are too long are considered weak, and muscles that are too short are considered strong in relation to each other.

Another way to look at weak and strong muscles is that any muscle that is too long or too short is weaker in relation to itself than it would be at a normal resting length. Optimal muscle strength happens when muscles are neither too long nor too short.

muscle homeostasis

The primary job of every system in the body, including the musculoskeletal system, is to maintain homeostasis. What this means is that each system is always making adjustments to maintain balance within the system.

When the muscular system is out of balance due to long periods of sitting or over/underuse, the muscles are constantly trying to get back into balance. This simply means that your system is trying to make your short muscles longer and your long muscles shorter. Here is an example: have you ever noticed that often when you are sitting in a chair, you have the urge to cross one leg over the other? This is quite common. It usually feels good. Even when we are told this is not good for us, we still do it. Why? Almost everybody has muscles that are too short on the outside of the upper leg and hip. Since your muscular system is trying to achieve balance (homeostasis), it feels comfortable when you cross one leg over the other, which gently stretches the short muscles on the outside of the leg and hip, making them longer. Your brain didn't make you do this; your body (muscular system) did. It is trying to show you how to bring your muscles back into balance.

Another example is when you lie down on your back. Many times you will notice that you find yourself automatically with both hands under your head. Again this usually feels good, and you didn't do it on purpose. Your muscular system made you do it. For most people, the muscles on the top of their shoulders are too long. When you put your hands under your head, you are shortening the muscles that are too long, helping them come back into balance.

When the muscular system imbalances are big enough, the body sends you a signal to do something about it. That signal is called pain. It is a call to bring your muscles back into balance.

important anatomical terms and key muscles

Use the following pages as a reference for key muscles and terms that will be useful in our study of asana. Eventually, these key muscles should be committed to memory in order to determine muscle imbalances. These muscles and anatomical terms are often mentioned in yoga classes.

It is not necessary to know all the individual names for the muscles. When appropriate, it is easier to refer to them by their actions, i.e. hip flexors, hip abductors, etc.

terms of movement

Flexion Moving in a way that decreases the angle at the joint (bending the joint).

Extension Moving in a way that increases the angle at the joint (straightening the joint).

Abduction Moving a limb away from the centerline of the body.

Adduction Moving a limb toward the centerline of the body.

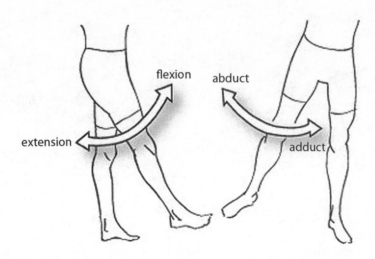

sections of the spine

Cervical Upper region of the spine usually referred to as C1–C7

Thoracic Middle region of the spine usually referred to as T1–T12

Lumbar Lower region of the spine usually referred to as L1–L5

regions of the body

Anterior Front side of the body

Posterior Backside of the body

Medial Toward the middle of the body

Lateral Toward the side of the body

muscle and bone parts

Ligament Attaches a bone to a bone

Tendon Attaches a muscle to a bone

Joint Where two bones meet

key muscles
hip flexors

Psoas

Quadriceps (Rectus femoris only)

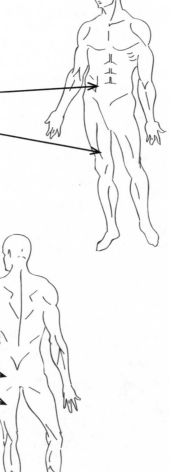

hip extensors

Gluteus maximus

Hamstrings

Semitendinosus

Semimembranosus

Biceps femoris

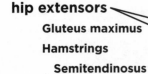

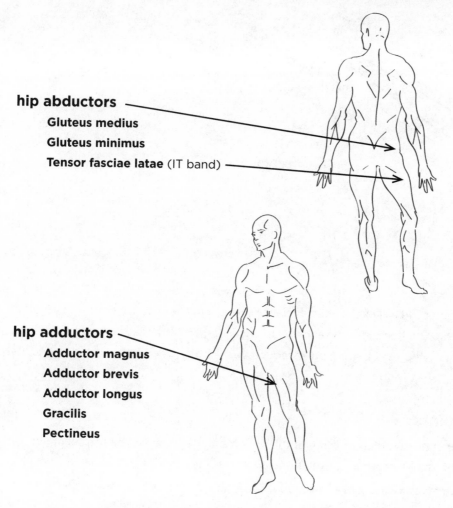

hip abductors
- Gluteus medius
- Gluteus minimus
- Tensor fasciae latae (IT band)

hip adductors
- Adductor magnus
- Adductor brevis
- Adductor longus
- Gracilis
- Pectineus

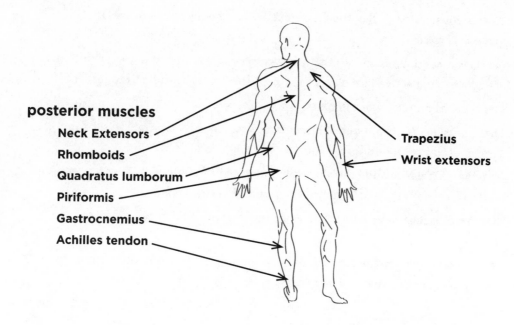

posterior muscles
- Neck Extensors
- Rhomboids
- Quadratus lumborum
- Piriformis
- Gastrocnemius
- Achilles tendon

Trapezius

Wrist extensors

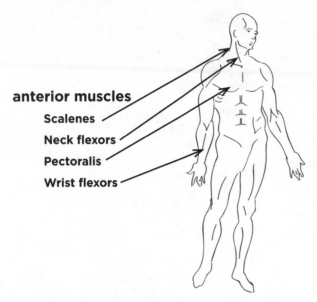

anterior muscles
    Scalenes
    Neck flexors
    Pectoralis
    Wrist flexors

In the next chapter, we will explore the ancient roots of yoga and discover that our modern practice is substantially different from the ancient practice. We will learn that the yoga we practice today is an excellent means to achieve a balanced, pain-free body when following the principles I will teach you.

Key Points

- **A basic understanding** of some of the systems in the body will be helpful in our study of asana—in particular the skeletal, fascial, nervous, and muscular systems.

- **The human body has 206 bones.** Ligaments connect these bones. The place where two bones meet is called a joint. Proper alignment of these bones is essential for optimal functioning.

- **The nervous system is like the electrical wiring in your house or car**. Its basic function is to send signals from one part of the body to others.

- **Fascia is a continuous sheath that runs from head to toe** without interruption. Also called connective tissue, it is the "glue" that holds everything together.

- **The skeletal muscles work in pairs.**

- **These muscles are often out of balance** due to over or underuse. This means some muscles become shorter, and some become longer.

- **Muscular imbalances pull the skeletal system out of alignment.** This can lead to nerve impingements, disc abnormalities, and fascial restrictions.

- **Optimal muscle strength** happens when muscles are neither too long nor too short.

- **When the muscle imbalances are big enough,** the body sends you a signal to do something about it. That signal is called pain.

CHAPTER 3

what is yoga? ancient and modern

"Yoga, an ancient but perfect science, deals with the evolution of humanity. This evolution includes all aspects of one's being, from bodily health to self-realization. Yoga means union—the union of body with consciousness and consciousness with the soul. Yoga cultivates the ways of maintaining a balanced attitude in day-to-day life and endows skill in the performance of one's actions."

—B.K.S. Iyengar

to understand how yoga can best be practiced today for well-being and pain relief, we must first recognize how yoga has changed since ancient times. The yoga that was practiced thousands of years ago in India is quite different than the yoga practiced around the world today. Many people falsely believe that the yoga as practiced today is an ancient form, developed by the yogic masters thousands of years ago. However, the original purpose of yoga was primarily as a spiritual practice with little focus on the poses. Today the opposite is true—we focus a great deal on the poses with little focus on the spiritual practice.

the original purpose of yoga

Among researchers, there is some debate as to when yoga was first developed. Some say five thousand years ago, and others say much more recently than that. Regardless of the age, yoga was originally designed as a spiritual discipline to achieve the union of ordinary consciousness and universal consciousness. This spiritual discipline was developed as a way to be able to lead a good life, by finding Ultimate Truth.

Traditionally, six paths of yoga lead toward this goal of finding Ultimate Truth; each one is a unique path leading to the same goal:

Karma Yoga - a form of yoga emphasizing the discipline of selfless action as a way to perfection.

> **Mantra Yoga** – a form of yoga that emphasizes the repetition of particular sounds representing a particular aspect of the Divine.
>
> **Bhakti Yoga** – a form of yoga emphasizing the spiritual practice of loving devotion to a personal form of the Divine.
>
> **Jnana Yoga** – a form of yoga emphasizing the path of knowledge as a way to the Divine.
>
> **Raja Yoga** – a form of yoga emphasizing control over the mind and emotions as a way to the Divine.
>
> **Hatha Yoga** – a form of yoga emphasizing a system of physical postures for balancing, stretching, and strengthening the body, the goal of which is to prepare the body for meditation.

The form of yoga most commonly practiced today is hatha yoga with its emphasis on the physical postures rather than meditation. Traditionally, yoga was more about meditation than the physical postures. In our modern world, the physical postures are emphasized, and instructors add some meditation and breathing exercises to the practice. However, the goal of all the types of yoga is to foster the union of body, mind, and spirit.

the eight limbs of yoga

Patanjali, whom scholars guess lived sometime in the second century BC, codified a system of finding this union of body, mind, and spirit in his work, the Yoga Sutras. This work is generally considered to be one of the foremost works on yoga.

Patanjali listed eight practices that serve as a comprehensive path that can lead us to the Divine. These are often known as the eight limbs of yoga. These limbs or practices apply to any of the six forms of yoga one has chosen to practice. They are designed to help quiet the mind. A quiet mind can then experience the higher states of consciousness and well-being. We will talk more about that in the chapter on meditation.

the eight limbs are:

Yama – Sanskrit for "moral discipline."

Niyama – Sanskrit for "moral observance."

These two practices deal with rules of behavior. They are the moral principles that help one to live a better life. These practices can be found in most every religion. Think The Ten Commandments or the Golden Rule.

Asana – Sanskrit for "seated posture."
This is the practice of sitting still and comfortable for meditation. The meaning of asana was later expanded to include stretching and strength training for flexibility and well-being. This limb of yoga is what we commonly practice today.

Pranayama – Sanskrit for "breath control."
This practice deals with the practice of breath control. Many different types of pranayama (breathing exercises) are used to regulate the life force (prana) of the body.

Pratyahara – Sanskrit for "withdrawal of the senses."
Stops the mind from reacting to sense perceptions.

Dharana – Sanskrit for "concentration."
Develops one pointed concentration for focus on the Divine.

Dhyana Sanskrit for "meditation."
The practice of mind control to stop thinking and come to realize the truth.

The three practices listed above bring the attention inward instead of outward to the physical world. The focus is on the inner world.

Samadhi – Sanskrit for "bliss" or "coming together into oneness.
This practice is the ultimate goal of yoga as understood originally.
Samadhi is becoming one with the divine.

Each one of these limbs is worthy of a separate book. They are practices that will help you in your search for the "best possible life. I encourage you to study these as part of your yoga practice, as they will benefit you in achieving your own greatness.

The original purpose of yoga, therefore, was to achieve union with the self and with God. It was designed to be a spiritual discipline. It is an all-encompassing system that can lead one to Self Realization and ultimately to God Realization.

As you can see from reading thus far, the original purpose of yoga was a spiritual practice that had a physical element—asana. Originally, asana referred only to the seated postures, as the ancient yogis were far more interested in meditation and God Realization. They needed to be comfortable in their seated posture so they could avoid the distractions of the body and focus on their meditation. The physical was one small part of this much bigger practice for achieving the blending of body, mind, and spirit. Asana was just one of the eight limbs.

the purpose of yoga as practiced today in the west

The yoga of today is very different than the yoga of the past. In the modern world, yoga is most often seen as a physical practice that has a spiritual element. When you mention yoga today, every-one immediately thinks of asana practice. It is interesting to note that the Sutras (often referred to as the Bible of yoga) mention little about asana practice. It is only mentioned in three places as far as I can see.

Hundreds of well-thought-out books have been written on asana practice and contain a lot of valuable information, and many more books are being written every year. This knowledge implies that from the time the Sutras were written until now, the practice of asana has evolved substantially to be far different than the ancient system. Ancient yoga was limited to mostly the seated postures. Today hundreds of poses are taught, each one having a particular benefit to the musculoskeletal system and the body as a whole. Many classes also include meditation and pranayama. A threefold approach to skillfully practicing asana, pranayama, and dhyana (medita-tion) can lead to a life free of stress and pain. It can lead to greater happiness and fulfillment. The research of today's modern science is now confirming more than ever the benefits of the above three practices.

modern asana practice

Mark Singleton has pointed out in his book *Yoga Body: The Origins of Modern Posture Practice* (2010, Oxford University Press) that modern yoga practice is substantially different from the ancient practice and has borrowed many of its ideas from European gymnastics and strength training. There is little evidence to support the theory that the ancient yogis practiced asana for health and fitness.

Furthermore, Nicholas Rosen, in his article "Going to the Mat: Confessions of a Yoga Guinea Pig" found that there is nothing ancient about the way we practice yoga today.

In a rare interview, BKS Iyengar, the 90-year old ambassador of yoga to the West, told me that his yoga, as taught to him by his master, was a purely physical exercise and completely unrelated to ancient philosophy. He says he invented and refined much of it himself. It wasn't until 1960, while on a visit to London, that English intellectuals introduced Iyengar to the ancient "yoga sutras." Five years later, he combined the yoga poses and the Hindu teachings together in his book "Light on Yoga," which then sold hundreds of thousands of copies in the United States. And voila—the modern yoga craze was born. But it was basically a new age invention, not an ancient practice.

"Going to the Mat: Confessions of a Yoga Guinea Pig" | Nicholas Rosen, http://www.huffingtonpost.com/nicholas-rosen/going-to-the-mat-confessi_b_186332.html (accessed December 3, 2014).

Although modern yoga is quite different than the practice of ancient yoga, this modern practice has many benefits and is worthy of pursuing, especially as an effective antidote to our culture of sitting. Yoga can also be extremely beneficial for many painful musculoskeletal conditions . . . if you are selecting the correct poses. Yoga also benefits our overworked nervous system, especially when we add pranayama and meditation to our practice. I also believe asana practice should keep evolving and become even better by learning more about the biomechanics of the muscular system and muscle physiology. This will help you understand how to select the correct poses to balance your body.

myth

Yoga is an ancient system of stretching developed thousands of years ago, so the postures I do in yoga class must be good for me.

fact

The poses that are popular in modern yoga classes have developed over the last one hundred years or so. They have their roots in gymnastics and strength training. It is essential that you select the correct pose for your current body condition to receive optimal results.

the benefits of modern yoga

If you already practice yoga, you know about the benefits this modern practice cultivates. You easily feel the value in your body. Yoga poses are especially beneficial when adding pranayama and meditation to your asana practice. These benefits are often divided into three categories—physical, mental, and spiritual.

Some of the physical benefits include:
• increased energy
• reduced pain
• increased flexibility
• improved circulation
• improved balance
• improved strength

Some of the mental benefits include:
• improved concentration
• reduced stress
• improved emotional states
• reduced anxiety
• increased body awareness

Some of the spiritual benefits include:
• increased sense of peace
• opening of the heart
• increased connection with the inner self
• increased sense of oneness with all of life

Of course, yoga provides many more benefits that I have not even mentioned. If yoga has evolved into a practice of mostly asana, based in gymnastics and strength training, more knowledge about the body and musculoskeletal system is required. It will require some knowledge of anatomy and the impact each asana will have on certain structures in the body.

balance your body, not your yoga practice

A widely held belief says that if you practice the postures diligently, yoga will bring agility, vitality, and balance. In my evaluations of thousands of yoga practitioners, I have found few who are in balance from a musculoskeletal point of view.

Balance can only be achieved if you are aware of your imbalances and restrictions and know which postures will be best suited for that condition. This knowledge will bring a more focused, aware practice. This practice will start to bring the body into balance and reduce or eliminate your pain. Like any discipline dealing with the musculoskeletal system, the muscles must be trained to be in balance. Failure to do so will result in pain.

I have been a yoga instructor for twenty years and a neuromuscular therapist for twenty-five years. Combining the knowledge contained in these two disciplines enables me to accurately choose which poses my body requires to become balanced and pain free. The knowledge I am sharing with you will help you understand why your hamstrings are still tight and why your hips won't open. I will explain to you why certain poses are difficult and even painful. Of course, I will also teach you how to correct those conditions.

Specifically, my approach will emphasize identifying muscle imbalances, choosing poses that will bring the musculoskeletal system into balance, and enhancing that experience with pranayama and meditation.

Modern yoga that is based in gymnastics can correct muscle imbalances in a relatively short time, but only if you learn to identify these imbalances and then practice the specific postures for those imbalances. Yoga has developed into a practice of performing poses. To achieve even greater benefit from your practice, the emphasis should be on selecting the correct pose that will bring the musculoskeletal system back into balance.

Performing yoga poses with an emphasis on correcting muscle imbalances instead of practicing poses will bring superior physical benefits. What is lacking in many yoga practices is the ability to evaluate and know which postures would be beneficial at this time for a particular body and the conditions it is presenting. There are hundreds of poses to choose from when practicing yoga. Learning and understanding the poses, and what muscles they are stretching or strengthening, will bring you the most benefit. Choosing the correct pose for your current muscle imbalances will result in the most therapeutic outcome.

Research has shown that when the muscles are in balance, many painful conditions are eliminated and range of motion increases. The body moves with more ease and grace. When the muscular system is in balance, the energetic life force (prana) flows better as well. This is one of the greatest benefits of asana practice.

Ask yourself the following questions every time you are practicing your yoga postures:

• Which muscles will I stretch today? Why?

• Which muscles will I strengthen today? Why?

• Which muscles will I neglect today? Why?

• Why did I choose a particular pose?

• What are my current muscle imbalances?

• Are the poses I selected the correct ones for my current imbalances?

• Who developed these poses and for what reason?

• Do you know?

• Does your teacher know?

If you cannot answer these questions, you are not receiving the maximum benefit from your yoga practice. You might be training your body to be out of balance.

As a neuromuscular therapist, I have treated many people for yoga injuries. The injuries are not because yoga is dangerous. Yoga is simply a tool. A tool does not make a mistake. It is the user of the tool who can make an error due to lack of knowledge that can cause harm. It is essential to know and recognize which postures to perform for a particular body condition and body type.

Some people have told me that they don't practice yoga because it is painful or is too difficult. Using my approach, yoga practice can be available to everyone regardless of their current physical condition or age. This is possible by following these general guidelines:

- The muscles must be trained slowly to come back into balance.

- Use a modified version of the pose, if necessary.

- Do not try to perform the full expression of a pose before the body is ready for it.

- Do not stretch into pain.

- Follow general alignment principles when performing poses, but the body does not necessarily benefit from doing the poses exactly the same way every time.

- The body benefits most by selecting the poses that will bring the body into balance and altering those poses for your current body condition.

Contrary to popular opinion, stretching a muscle is not always good for it. Neither does practicing poses with correct alignment automatically bring the body into balance. Many yoga teachers have intuitively figured this out but do not know why.

Having a good background in anatomy is a useful tool. However, even if you don't have this knowledge, I will show you how you can quickly look at your body and determine where the muscular imbalances are and how to know exactly which poses to select. I assure you it is not as difficult as you might imagine. It is not even necessary to know the names of all the muscles, although that can be useful.

meditation and pranayama

Adding meditation and pranayama to your yoga practice will bring even better overall health and well-being to the body, mind, and spirit. The ancient yogis did not separate asana, pranayama, and meditation. They considered it all one practice. Asana was practiced to balance the body, pranayama to balance the nervous system, and meditation to balance the brain. These practices, which we will discuss in more depth in chapters 11 and 12, will relax the muscles and calm the nervous system even more than just practicing asana. They will reward you with an energized body, a calm nervous system, and a clear, focused mind that will reduce stress and anxiety. This threefold approach to yoga brings superior results. Meditation and pranayama are as relevant today as they were in ancient times.

In the next chapter, we will receive a better understanding of what the postures are stretching or strengthening. If we are to have a more beneficial practice, this knowledge will be essential. We will break down the poses into five groups, some of which overlap: front folds, back bends, side bends, twists, and hip openers.

Key Points:

- **Yoga was first developed** as a spiritual practice.

- **The ultimate goal** was union with God through meditation.

- **Yoga has eight branches or limbs.** Seven deal with the spiritual. One—asana— deals with the physical.

- **Asana was developed to help the body sit comfortably** in meditation.

- **Yoga as practiced today is mainly a physical practice.** It is derived from gymnastics and strength training.

- **Understanding basic musculoskeletal anatomy** is the key to keeping the muscles in balance and receiving the most benefit from your practice.

- **What is lacking** in many yoga practices is the ability to evaluate and know which postures would be beneficial at this time, for a particular body and the conditions it is presenting.

- **My approach to yoga** will emphasize identifying muscle imbalances, choosing poses that will bring the musculoskeletal system into balance, and enhancing that experience with pranayama and meditation.

- **Performing yoga poses** with an emphasis on correcting muscle imbalances, instead of practicing poses, will bring superior physical benefits.

- **Yoga can correct muscle imbalances** in a relatively short time only if you learn to identify these imbalances and then practice the specific postures for those imbalances.

- **A body in balance has little to no pain.**

- **Practicing meditation and pranayama** will help reduce stress and anxiety and will enhance your asana practice by relaxing muscles.

choosing the correct postures to achieve muscle balance

"The body benefits most when the postures are performed consciously and with full understanding. It takes time to accomplish difficult postures. Avoid forcing the body into them prematurely. Work into them gradually. Otherwise, the body can be harmed."

—Swami Kripalu

How can you know which postures are most beneficial for your current body condition? Which poses will help with your current painful condition or imbalance? Which poses will aggravate your condition? The ability to answer these questions is the key to getting the maximum benefit from your practice.

Modern yoga postures (asanas) are primarily based on nineteenth-century British gymnastics, not on two-thousand-year-old traditions. They are designed to lengthen and strengthen muscles, which is what the body needs for balance and health. Modern yoga's orientation toward a balanced practice relates to achieving a balance among the major categories of asana—forward bends, backward bends, side bends, twists, and hip openers—rather than achieving a balanced body. Thus, imbalances in the body are often aggravated by the typical modern yoga practice.

Yoga has developed into a practice of performing poses. The objective should be selecting the correct pose that will bring the musculoskeletal system back into balance. Each pose should be looked at as a tool for accomplishing the goal of a balanced body.

I am often asked what is the best form of yoga to practice. Should I be practicing hot yoga, yin yoga, restorative yoga, or some other type? My answer is the type of yoga you do is not nearly as important as selecting the correct poses for your current musculoskeletal condition.

In every posture, some muscles are made longer and some muscles are made shorter. We need a better understanding of what each asana is stretching or strengthening if we are to have a more beneficial practice. For our study of asana, it will be beneficial to break down the poses into five groups, some of which overlap:

- Front folds
- Back bends
- Side bends
- Twists
- Hip openers

Front folds are postures that involve bending forward at the waist. In general, these postures are stretching muscles on the backside of the body and strengthening muscles on the front side.

Back bends are postures that involve bending backward at the waist. In general, these postures stretch the front side of the body and strengthen muscles on the backside.

Side bends are postures that involve bending the body to one side. In general, these postures stretch one side of the body and strengthen the other side.

Twists are postures that involve rotating the body to one side. In general, these postures stretch the muscles on the outside of the thigh and the muscles along the spine and strengthen the inside of the thigh.

Hip openers are postures that involve bringing the legs away from the body. In general, these postures stretch the inside of the thigh and strengthen the outside of the thigh. In the typical chair-sitting body, the muscles on the front of the body and the muscles on the outside hip are usually too short. The muscles on the back of the body (except the calf) and the muscles of the inside thigh are usually too long. These muscle imbalances are the primary cause of many neuromuscular conditions.

Armed with this knowledge, we can begin to see that it will be more beneficial to focus on stretching muscles that are too short and strengthening muscles that are too long (strengthening a muscle makes it shorter). This implies that most of us should start by practicing mostly twists, side bends, and back bends until our bodies start to come back into balance. Front folds and hip openers should be practiced sparingly in the beginning or not at all depending on the severity of your condition.

the myth of a balanced practice

Do you have a balanced practice?

Should you have a balanced practice?

In the practice of asana, balance is the most important aspect of your practice. Most people in the yoga community talk about a balanced practice, but I don't think I can ever remember somebody actually executing a balanced practice. If you think about all the yoga classes you have participated in, is it not true that 60–70% of the class was spent practicing forward folds and hip openers? That certainly is not a balanced practice. Even worse, these forward folds and hip openers are stretching muscles that are too long in almost everybody. By emphasizing these poses over others, muscle imbalances can be exacerbated.

A balanced practice would put equal emphasis on the five groups of poses. This would stretch all the muscle groups equally. At first, that sounds like a good idea. But, let's think about that a bit. In my years as a neuromuscular therapist, I have seen few bodies that were in balance or even close to being in balance.

If the vast majority of people are out of balance and they have a balanced practice (stretching all the muscle groups equally), this would keep the body out of balance. To bring the body back into balance, you need to focus only on stretching the muscles that are too short for a period of time. This practice could take three to five months, not long considering how long you have been out of balance. Once your muscles are in balance, then a balanced practice is a right course of action. By changing one's thinking and learning to balance the body rather than the practice itself, you can achieve better health for yourself and your yoga students.

myth

If I perform hip openers, my hips will become more flexible.

fact

Hip openers will open the front of your hips but will make the side and the back of the hips even tighter.

Yoga can correct these muscle imbalances in a relatively short time only if you learn to identify these imbalances and then practice the specific postures for those imbalances. Don't worry! I am going to help you figure this all out in a simple, straightforward manner.

Your yoga practice can be deceptive because initially you will feel better. You feel better because the stretching is bringing increased blood and oxygen to the tissues. When you feel better, you continue the same practice. What happens is that, at some point, because you did not know how to recognize muscle imbalances, you start to develop some aches and pains or maybe some restricted range of motion. What happened? You made your muscle imbalances more pronounced by choosing the wrong pose for your current body condition. Varying your routine is important.

does it make any sense to stretch muscles that are too long?

Yes, it is beneficial to stretch muscles that are too long with the caveat that they should only be stretched slightly and not too often. The intention is to bring some blood, oxygen, and prana to these tissues. I call that waking up the muscles.

what are the best poses for me?

If you look on the Internet, you will find many suggestions for which yoga poses will give you the greatest benefit. It seems everyone has a different opinion. You will often hear that forward folds are calming, and that inverted poses are good for headaches, and so on. Usually, a good reason is not given as to why these poses are the best. This "formula" approach to yoga can lead to poor results. Also, poses are often recommended that are not accessible to many people, given their current muscular imbalances. This is one of the reasons more people are not practicing yoga.

The typical chair-sitting Western body should start doing more back bends, twists, and side bends. These poses target muscles that are usually too short. Many people do not like these poses as much as the hip openers and front folds because they are typically more difficult. These muscles that you have been making short your whole life will take some time to elongate and come back into balance. It is imperative that we start using more of these poses. They will need to be modified or supported with props until the full expression of the pose becomes available.

Front bends and hip openers can be practiced with the caveat that you not stretch them deeply. It is a matter of intention. Short muscles require a more sustained, deeper (but not too deep) stretch than long muscles. Once your muscles come into balance, you can spend equal amounts of time on the various groups of poses.

Knowing which muscles to strengthen is also valuable. The poses that strengthen muscles on the back of the body and the inner thigh are most beneficial when trying to bring the body into balance. Bridge pose (while squeezing a block between your knees) will strengthen the hamstrings, the gluteals, the rhomboids, and the adductors. It is a good place to start, as that pose will strengthen several muscle groups that are typically too long.

don't be afraid to modify the postures for your condition

Yoga is called a practice. You need to practice to achieve the pose. Many people try to perform the full expression of the pose before their body is ready for it. This will often lead to injury and frustration. Many of the poses in this book will come with a modification so they are accessible to all body types and conditions. Do not try to force the body open. Start with a modification and, through practice, the full expression of the pose then becomes available.

I have noticed in yoga class that if the teacher modifies a pose, the students will adjust. If the teacher talks about a modification but doesn't do the modification, students usually won't do it either.

As a yoga practitioner, you should not hesitate to modify a pose if that feels better to you. You should not try to do the full expression of the pose if it is causing pain. Many yoga students try to push through the pain. I do not believe that is a good idea. Pain is your body giving you a clear message to stop. If you stretch too deeply, you start to elongate the attachment points. That is not ideal. You want to stretch in the midrange of that muscle. Stretching in the midrange brings better, longer-lasting results.

Modifying the poses for your current imbalance is wise, as is using a full range of props. Props should include straps, blocks, blankets, cushions, and anything else that will help you safely stretch your target muscle without pain.

contraindications

A contraindication refers to a situation where a specific pose might be harmful to a particular person based on their health and current muscle imbalances. In general, if you experience pain while practicing a pose, that is a contraindication.

As yoga has become more popular, injury rates have been steadily rising. It is imperative that yoga teachers and yoga students become more aware of the contraindications as it relates to their situation.

pain

Pain is the first and most visible signal of a contraindication to the pose being performed. This is usually due to stretching too deeply or stretching a muscle that is already too long. Modifying that pose will usually solve that issue. Pain could also be the result of a current medical condition. Never stretch into pain. Humans are the only species that stretch into pain. Listening to your body when practicing asanas means you should not stretch into pain.

medical conditions

Some standard medical conditions warrant particular attention when practicing yoga:

- Recent surgeries

- Hip and knee replacements

- Joint issues like severe arthritis

- Cardiac conditions

- High or low blood pressure

- Glaucoma

- Pregnancy

- Disc abnormalities

Before practicing yoga, make sure to consult with a doctor if you have or suspect that you have any of the above conditions. Once the doctor clears you, make sure your yoga teacher knows about your conditions as well.

guidelines for maximum benefit from your practice

- Warm up the muscles before stretching.

- Park your ego at the door and practice with a more mindful intention. Yoga is not a sport or competition.

- Do not stretch more than 75% of what you think you are capable of stretching.
- Do not struggle in a posture. Yoga should not be painful. Make appropriate use of props to support you.
- Limit front folds and hip openers until your muscles come back into balance.
- Add a few more back bends and twists, which often target the muscles that are too short.
- Use your breath to ease into the posture.
- Hold each posture as long as it is comfortable and work up to 1–3 minutes.
- Vary your routine. Students often keep doing the same practice over and over. This is a not a good idea. The body and the muscles will adapt to your routine, and your practice will plateau.

In the next chapter, we will look at the importance of stretching correctly. How to stretch is often more important than what to stretch. Learning the basics of muscle stretching will take your practice to the next level.

Key Points

- **We need a full understanding** of what the postures are stretching or strengthening if we are to have a more beneficial practice.
- **Yoga has developed into a practice of performing poses.** The objective should be selecting the correct pose that will bring the musculoskeletal system back into balance. Each pose should be viewed as a tool for accomplishing the goal of a balanced body.
- **Breaking down the poses into five groups,** some of which overlap, is beneficial: front folds, back bends, side bends, twists, hip openers.
- **By focusing on stretching the short muscles,** you can bring the body back into balance. This could take three to five months.
- **Until our muscles come back into balance,** we should focus on twists, side bends, and back bends.
- **Stretch muscles that are too long** with the caveat that they should only be stretched slightly and not too often.
- **Varying your routine is important.**
- **Some standard medical conditions warrant particular attention** when practicing yoga. Consult your doctor before practicing yoga.

CHAPTER 5

the dangers of overstretching

"Do not kill the instinct of the body for the glory of the pose."

——Vanda Scaravelli

Now that we have learned how muscle imbalances can cause discomfort in the body, we must learn how to correct those imbalances. In chapters 6 through 10 we will discuss which muscles to stretch to correct particular imbalances. However, the first skill we need to acquire is learning how to stretch. If we don't stretch properly, we are setting ourselves up for a poor result. Improper stretching is one of the reasons people go to yoga class and never come back!

Stretching provides many benefits, including greater flexibility, increased joint range of motion, improved circulation, better posture, and less stress. All these benefits will make you feel better. Sometimes, however, you don't feel better. You might even get injured. How can this happen?

Two factors will increase the risk of being injured in yoga—stretching the wrong muscles and stretching the muscles too deeply. People often strive to perform the full expression of a pose before the body is ready. Remember that asana practice should not be about practicing poses. It should be about selecting the poses that will bring the body back into balance. The glory is not in achieving a particular pose. The glory is a balanced, pain-free body. When you are stretching muscles, you are also stretching all the other soft, connective tissue as well, including fascia, tendons, and ligaments. Stretching tendons and ligaments is generally not a good idea unless you have a good reason to do so.

Sports MDs have observed that many injuries in yoga are from repetitive strain, pushing too hard to achieve a pose and not listening to the body. They further state that they have seen many hip injuries that lead to osteoarthritis and eventually to hip replacements.

Stretching should feel good. If you watch a cat or a dog stretch, you will see that they experience no strain and that they look happy and relaxed. When you watch people stretch, you will often notice that they look strained, and they are working hard. What is the difference between animals and people when it comes to stretching? Animals are listening to their bodies. People are listening to their brains. The human brain keeps telling us if a little stretch feels good, a bigger stretch is even better. This mistake will often lead to pain.

My observations as a therapist for twenty-five years have shown that bringing muscles back into balance requires only consistent, moderate stretches that feel good. If you have soreness the next day, or if the stretch you are performing is painful, you probably overstretched your muscles. This is especially true if you have stretched a muscle that was already too long.

Remember that yoga is not a sport. Trying to do the full expression of a pose before the body is ready or because it is the wrong pose for your current muscle imbalances can cause many painful conditions. We are often instructed in yoga class to go to the edge and hold the pose. The truth is you will receive a better benefit from the stretch if you stretch no more than 75%! This will stretch the middle of the muscle and not put stress on the ends of the muscle where they attach.

I have not told you yet, but I am also a professional trumpet player. I have been playing for forty years. I had to practice to become proficient on my instrument. I could not play the full expression of a song for at least ten years. My body had not yet acquired enough training and skill. I find it interesting that in yoga class, students are trying to do the full expression of a pose after a month or two. More training and practice is required before trying to stretch into the full pose. Not pushing the body to do a full expression of a pose before it is ready is most prudent.

myth

The goal of asana practice is to be able to perform the full expression of the pose.

fact

Yoga is not about performing poses. It is about wisely choosing which poses (stretches) will be best for your current body imbalances and conditions and to only stretch as far as the body will comfortably allow you.

Whenever I treat someone for an injury that happened in yoga class, I always ask what pose they were doing when they got hurt. Ninety-five percent of the time they were injured doing a pose that was stretching an overstretched muscle. In other words, stretching a short muscle seldom causes an injury.

understanding fascia

In chapter 2, I gave you a definition of fascia. This would be a good time to go back and review it to make it clearer in your mind. Fascia is often referred to as soft tissue or connective tissue. Fascia interpenetrates the muscles. Muscle and fascia are not separate systems; they are woven together. You cannot stretch muscle without stretching fascia. Fascia, like muscles, can develop restrictions that are painful and/or compromise your range of motion.

The most important fact you need to know about fascia is that it responds to a stretch differently than muscle. Muscle responds to a firm stretch lasting thirty seconds or so. Fascia requires a gentle, low intensity stretch of one minute or more. If you are stretching your muscles for thirty seconds, your fascia may not be receiving the stretch it needs to clear its restrictions. Start by holding your poses thirty seconds and work up to one minute or more. This will give your muscles and the fascia enough time to stretch.

signs of overstretching

The biggest challenge I face as a yoga teacher is trying to convince my students not to stretch too deeply. I have observed that some of my students actually enjoy the pain they receive from stretching! Many people are not able to determine if they are stretching too deeply. As a rule of thumb, if you feel like saying ouch, or you really want to come out of that pose now, you are stretching too deeply.

There are usually clues the body gives us to let us know we are stretching too often or too deeply. While there may be many signs, some of the most prominent are:

- The hamstrings ache all the time, especially behind the knee or at the ischial tuberosity (sitz bones).
- The hip adductors ache, especially in the groin area or the medial side of the knee.
- The low back hurts or radiates pain down the leg. This includes SI joint pain and sacrum pain.
- The muscle you are stretching hurts.
- The joint above or below the muscle you are stretching hurts.
- The opposing muscle on the other side of the body cramps.

No pain, no gain does not apply to stretching;
it only applies to weight training.

what is the stretch reflex?

In simple terms, the stretch reflex should be thought of as the muscles' built-in protection mechanism. It helps the body to maintain balance and protects it from injury. Any stretch will activate the stretch reflex, which will cause the muscle that is being stretched to contract—**the deeper and more forceful the stretch, the greater the contraction.** The body senses that this forceful movement might cause a muscle to tear, and by contracting, the muscle is less likely to tear. If you continue to stretch too deeply, you will override the stretch reflex, likely resulting in some painful condition.

Let's take a closer look at some of the problems associated with overstretching.

muscle tears

When you stretch too deeply, you are putting abnormal stress on the muscles that can lead to a tear. A muscle tear can manifest as a micro tear, a substantial tear or even a complete tear. In any case, you will feel some sensation of pain and/or bruising. These symptoms usually show up the next day. At this point, you may think that being sore the next day is a good sign and that you should keep stretching that muscle until the pain goes away. This is not a good idea. Overstretching a muscle can cause it to tear.

strained tendons and sprained ligaments

Stretching too deeply can lead to strained tendons and sprained ligaments.

A tendon is a dense band of tissue that attaches muscle to a bone. An example is the Achilles tendon that attaches the calf muscle to the heel bone. Touch your Achilles tendon and notice how dense it feels in relation to the calf muscle itself. A strain is an overstretch or tear in the muscle or tendon.

A ligament is a dense band of tissue that attaches a bone to another bone across a joint. Ligaments cross all the joints in the body. An example is the anterior cruciate ligament (ACL) that attaches the femur to the tibia at the knee. A sprain is an overstretch or tear in the ligament.

Both of these injuries can lead to joint instability.

muscle weakness and joint dysfunction

Muscles that are consistently overstretched lead to muscle weakness and joint dysfunction (instability). An example of this is the imbalance between the hamstrings on the back of the upper thigh and the quadriceps on the front side of the upper thigh; most people present with long, overstretched, weak hamstrings and short, strong quads. This imbalance will result in a forward tilt to the pelvis that may cause the sacroiliac joint (SI joint) in the low back to become unstable and often painful.

inflammation

Overstretching can lead to pain and inflammation in the soft tissues themselves or in the joints. Symptoms of inflammation include redness, swelling, heat, and pain. An example would be Achilles tendonitis. Some of the latest research has indicated that inflammation is not part of the problem but is actually the body's response to a condition and is part of the healing process. In any case, inflammation is a sign of a problem.

how to stretch for maximum benefit

- Warm up the muscles before stretching. This means you have to make the muscles warmer by raising the body temperature at least one degree. This warmup should include some type of aerobic activity and some joint rotations. This should take ten to fifteen minutes. Muscles stretch better when they are warm.

- Identify which muscles are too long and which muscles are too short. In both cases, they might feel tight. Common muscle groups that are too long are the hamstrings, the adductors, and the rhomboids. Common muscle groups that are too short are the pectoral muscles, the psoas, and the quadriceps.

- If a muscle is too short, set the intention that you are going to make it longer. Stretch those muscles to 75% or less of your maximum effort. Muscles respond better to a stretch in the midrange than at their end range.

- If a muscle is too long, set your intention to "wake the muscle up" but not try to make it longer. By this I mean stretch the muscle a little (25%) to bring more blood and oxygen to it, but the intention is not to make it longer by stretching deeply.

- Hold each posture for at least one minute, but make sure you are not straining in the pose. Holding the stretch longer will stretch both the fascia and the muscles. If you cannot hold the posture for a minute, you are stretching too deeply.

- Make appropriate use of props to support you. Do not struggle in a posture; modify if necessary. Props may include blocks, straps, blankets, and cushions. They will help you achieve a better result.

- Do not bounce in a stretch. This can lead to muscle tears.

- Use your breath to ease into the posture. We will talk about this more in chapter 11.

- Park your ego at the door and practice with a more mindful intention. Do not stretch more than 75% of what you think you are capable of stretching. This practice is about doing what is right for your body. It does not matter what the guy next to you is doing!

We are now ready to start correcting muscle imbalances. In the next chapter we will learn how to correct muscle imbalances using modern yoga poses. We will begin with the five major imbalances.

Key Points

- **Knowing how to stretch** is as important as knowing what to stretch.

- **Stretching should feel good, not painful.**

- **Two factors that contribute to injuries** in yoga are stretching the wrong muscles for your current condition and stretching too deeply.

- **If you have soreness the next day,** or if the stretch you are performing is painful, you probably overstretched your muscles.

- **Trying to do the full expression of a pose** before the body is ready or because it is the wrong pose for your current muscle imbalances can cause many painful conditions.

- **Overstretching can cause muscle tears,** strained tendons, sprained ligaments, muscle weakness, and inflammation.

- **Bringing muscles into balance requires** only moderate, consistent stretches.

- **Warm up muscles before stretching them.**

- **Muscles and fascia require a stretch of at least one minute** to start to unwind.

- **Do not stretch more than 75%.**

- **Use your breath** to ease into a stretch.

CHAPTER 6

achieving muscular/skeletal balance

*"Once your foundation is improved, it is much easier
to put the rest of your house in order."*
—Leslie Kaminoff, Yoga Anatomy, Second Edition

In this chapter, I will show you how to correct the five major muscle imbalances using common poses (stretches/strengthenings) that will serve as the foundation for your practice. Being intentional and present will bring the best results.

Correcting muscle imbalances is not nearly as difficult as it might sound. The muscles will do exactly what you train them to do. Stretching will make a muscle longer, and strengthening will make a muscle shorter. It is simply a matter of stretching muscles that are too short and strengthening muscles that are too long. When done consistently, you can bring your body back into balance in three to five months. Sometimes it will take a little longer.

Remember the questions that are essential to ask yourself when practicing yoga.

• Which muscles did I stretch today? Why?

• Which muscles did I strengthen today? Why?

• Which muscles did I neglect today? Why?

• Why did I choose a particular pose?

• Are the poses I selected the correct ones for my current imbalances?

When you view the body in terms of muscular imbalances, the above questions become easier to answer. Deciding which poses you will do becomes much easier, and more importantly, you will know why you are stretching certain muscles and strengthening others. You will also realize that you typically stretch or ignore the same muscles in every practice.

focus on the five major imbalances

Recognizing muscle imbalances is essential to take yoga and your practice to the next level. This endeavor is not nearly as difficult as one might expect. You will be on your way to better posture and less pain when you learn to identify and correct the five major imbalances. If corrected, most of the smaller imbalances will fall into place. Once you know what to look for, it is pretty obvious.

correct the cause, not the symptom

The site of pain in the body is not necessarily where the pain is originating. For example, many cases of low back pain are caused by tight, short muscles on the front side of the body known as the hip flexors. (We identified the hip flexors in chapter 2.) This pain can often be deceiving, as the hip flexors don't hurt but the low back hurts a lot.

When dealing with low back pain, many people immediately think they need to be stretching their back. While this is often true, this course of action will only bring temporary, symptomatic relief because the cause has not yet been addressed.

To achieve more long-lasting relief, all the muscle imbalances need to be addressed, not just the site of the pain.

which muscles should I be stretching?

If you want to get the maximum benefit out of your yoga practice and not injure yourself, you should mainly stretch the muscles that are too short.

Fortunately, most people have the same muscle imbalances because we all do similar things like sit in a car or at a computer. To review, muscles on the front of the body are too short and muscles on the back of the body are too long except for the calves. Muscles on the outside of the thigh are generally too short and on the inside of the thigh too long. Remember, the muscles that are too long most often feel much tighter than the short ones.

To review, stretching muscles that are too long is OK with the caveat that these should not be the main focus, and you should not strive to stretch them too deeply.

We should focus our stretching on the front and side of the body and the outside of the thigh. This means mainly back bends, sidebends, and twists. When your muscles start to come back into balance, then you can add in the other postures.

which muscles should i be strengthening?

There are benefits to strengthening all the muscles in your body. However muscles on the backside of the body (other than the calves) and muscles on the inside of the thigh are typically too long in the average chair-sitting body. These muscles should be primarily strengthened. Strengthening a muscle will make it shorter over time and will bring the body back into balance. Several yoga poses can accomplish this goal, which I will show you later in the book.

align the pelvis

The key to muscular skeletal balance is first to align the pelvis. The pelvis serves as the foundation for the rest of the body structure. To illustrate this principle, think of a house on a concrete foundation. If the foundation starts to sink a little bit on one end, it will in turn make the structure of the entire house malaligned, resulting in abnormal stress on the structure. By starting with the pelvis, we set a solid foundation on which to build. When the pelvis comes into balance, many other muscle imbalances in the upper and lower body are also corrected.

correcting the three major pelvic imbalances

There are three predominate pelvic imbalances—elevated pelvis, rotated pelvis, and tilted pelvis. Many people present with all three pelvic imbalances in varying degrees. Some may be more rotated, tilted, or elevated, but even one of these imbalances can be the source of many painful neuromuscular conditions. Many of these imbalances are caused by improper sitting positions. Let's look at how we are able to correct these muscle imbalances and bring the body back into alignment.

elevated pelvis

An elevated pelvis looks like one hip is higher than the other. This condition is quite common and is caused by muscle imbalances (unless there is a bone length discrepancy, which is rare). The difference can be anywhere from a fraction of an inch to two inches or more. This also means one leg is shorter than the other—not truly short as in a bone length difference but functionally short when you are walking.

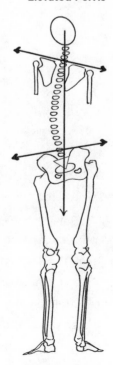

Elevated Pelvis

This condition often occurs when the quadratus lumborum muscle in the low back is too short on one side. The action of this muscle is to hike up the hip. Sometimes it is locked short on one side, causing the pelvis to elevate on that side, which can then cause scoliosis.

An elevated pelvis could also lead to abnormal strain on the hip and knee joints, improper gait, and abnormal strain on the lumbar discs. I have observed that many times the pain from an elevated pelvis is on the side with the longer leg, not the shorter. An elevated pelvis also contributes to a rotated pelvis.

testing for an elevated pelvis

It is difficult to measure yourself to see if you have an elevated pelvis, but it is easy if you have a friend who will assist you.

- Lie down on your back.
- Have your friend lightly grasp your ankles and gently lean back, giving you a little traction.

• Locate the two ankle bones (malleoli) on the inside of each ankle and have the friend place their thumbs on each bone. These are the "bumps" on the inside of the ankle.

• Bring the legs together in the middle of the body and see if the ankle bones line up. Sometimes they do, but usually they don't.

The leg with the higher ankle bone is the short one.

correcting an elevated pelvis

You can start to correct an elevated pelvis by stretching the quadratus lumborum muscle in the low back. Standing Crescent Moon Pose will target this muscle. Since you cannot measure yourself, you should do this stretch on both sides. Consistent stretching of this muscle will bring the elevated pelvis back down to a more neutral position. It is a good idea to do this on a daily basis. Do this pose morning and evening for one minute.

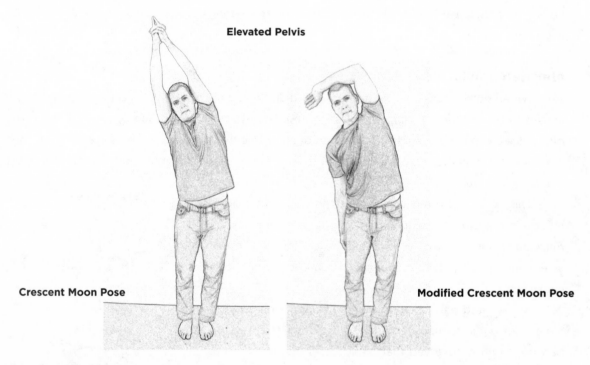

Elevated Pelvis

Crescent Moon Pose

Modified Crescent Moon Pose

rotated pelvis

A rotated or twisted pelvis is when one hip is more forward than the other hip. This condition is often due to muscle imbalances pulling on one side of the hip in relation to the other side. This will often present as short external rotators deep in the buttocks (think piriformis) and short abductors (think IT band) on the outside thigh. The condition can cause a jammed SI joint in the low back. The SI joint is where the sacrum meets the iliac crest. A rotated pelvis could also lead to abnormal strain on the hip and knee joints, improper gait, and abnormal strain on the lumbar discs. A rotated pelvis also contributes to an elevated pelvis.

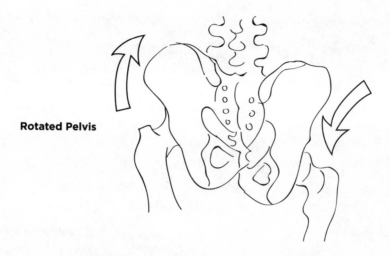

Rotated Pelvis

testing for a rotated pelvis

Lie down on your back and completely relax. Observe the position of your legs. Do they turn out? Most people think this is normal because this is the way everyone looks. Make sure you are looking at your legs and not your feet, as some people's ankles turn in. When your legs are externally rotated, that internally rotates the pelvis on that side and may externally rotate it on the other side.

A quick note here: It is OK for your legs to turn out for twenty minutes while you are in deep relaxation pose (Savasana). It is not so good if they are turned out for twenty years.

correcting a rotated pelvis

You can correct a rotated pelvis by stretching the piriformis muscle deep in the buttocks and the abductor muscles located on the outer thigh. Supine Twist Pose will target these muscles. It will also be helpful to strengthen the adductor muscle group on the inside of the thigh. Consistent stretching of the abductors and piriformis combined with consistent strengthening of the adductors starts to bring the pelvis out of its rotation. Practice this stretch three to four times a day.

To strengthen the adductors, place a pillow between your knees and squeeze the knees together ten times for three seconds each time. Do three sets of these twice a day.

It may take three to five months to retrain the muscles and correct the rotation.

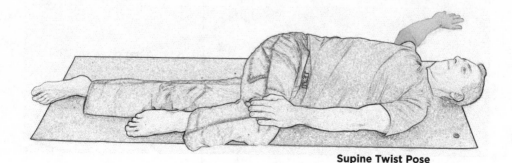

Supine Twist Pose

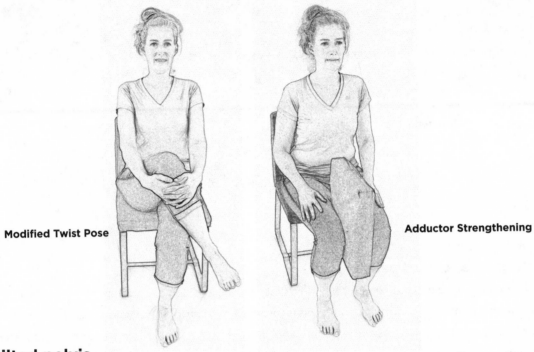

Modified Twist Pose

Adductor Strengthening

tilted pelvis

A forward (anterior) tilt to the pelvis occurs when the hip flexor muscles (psoas and rectus femoris) are too short and they pull the pelvis forward. The result is an exaggerated curve in the low back. This is a common muscle imbalance.

The most prominent symptom of short hip flexors is low back pain.

A tilted pelvis can also lead to abnormal strain on the hip and knee joints, improper gait, and abnormal strain on the lumbar discs and SI joint.

A backward (posterior) tilt to the pelvis occurs when the hip extensor muscles (gluteus maximus and hamstrings) are too short. This condition is very rare. Most people present with a forward (anterior) tilt.

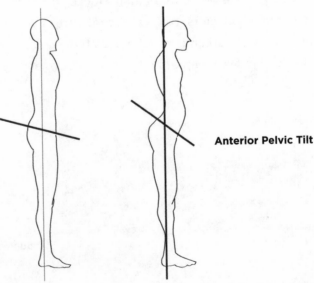

Anterior Pelvic Tilt

testing for an anterior tilt

To test if tight hip flexor muscles are causing your low back pain, lie down flat on your back and completely relax. This position will often make your back feel worse after a while. Then bend your knees so that your feet are flat on the mat. This will take the strain off the quadriceps and psoas (hip flexors). Does that make your back feel better? If it did, then you have short, tight hip flexors. To be a little more specific, when lying on your back, is there a gap between the low back and the floor? The bigger the gap, the shorter the psoas. When lying on your back, is there a gap under your knees? If there is, you have a short, tight rectus femoris muscle (quad).

correcting an anterior tilt

You can correct a forward tilted pelvis by stretching the quad muscles on the front of the thigh and the psoas muscles deep in the core. This version of Pigeon Pose will target these muscles. Pigeon Pose may be too deep of a stretch for some people, so I have also given you some off-the-mat stretches that will target the quads and psoas.

Strengthening the gluteal muscles and the hamstring muscles on the back of the thigh is also helpful. Consistent stretching of the quads and psoas combined with consistent strengthening of the hamstrings and gluteal muscles starts to bring the pelvis out of its forward tilt. This stretch should be practiced three to four times a day for at least one minute each time.

To strengthen the hamstrings and gluteal muscles, you can perform Bridge Pose. Practice this pose three times a day. Start with thirty seconds if you can, and work up to two minutes. Make sure the pose is not painful; you don't want to put further strain on the back.

It may take three to five months to retrain the muscles and correct the tilt.

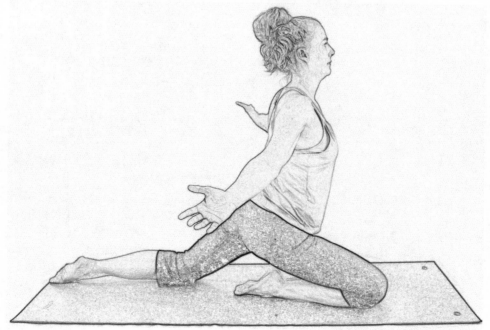

Pigeon Pose

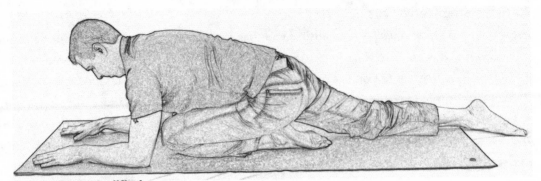

Pigeon Pose Modified

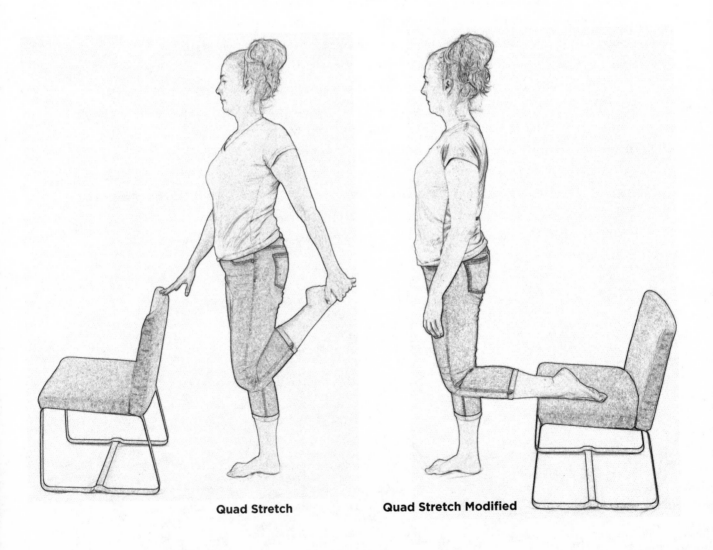

Quad Stretch   **Quad Stretch Modified**

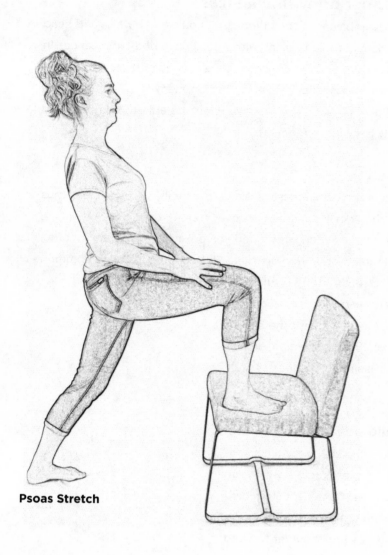

Psoas Stretch

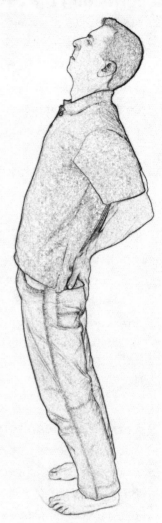

Psoas Stretch Modified

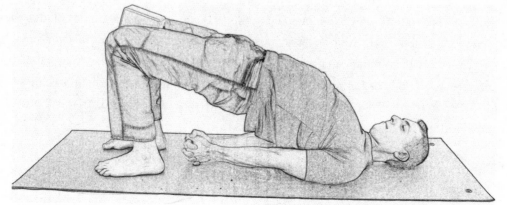

Bridge Pose with block between knees

correcting the two major upper body imbalances

There are two predominate upper body imbalances—head forward/shoulders forward, and head tilted to the side/elevated shoulder. Many people present with both upper body imbalances in varying degrees. Some may be more forward, tilted, or elevated, but even one of these imbalances can be the source of many painful neuromuscular conditions. In my opinion, many of these imbalances are caused by improper sitting positions. Let's look at how we might be able to correct these muscle imbalances and bring the body back into alignment.

head forward/ shoulders forward

Head forward/shoulders forward occurs when the chest muscles (pectorals) are too short, thus pulling the rhomboids between the shoulder blades into an overstretched position. When the head goes forward (for example, when you are sitting improperly or looking down at your phone), the shoulders will round forward and the chest will look sunken. This condition is quite common and most likely due to a lifetime of incorrectly sitting in chairs.

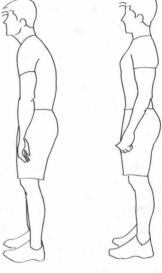

Head forward/shoulders forward can lead to abnormal strain on the cervical discs. This could lead to headaches, brain fog, jaw pain, shoulder pain, neck pain, and restrictions in the range of motion in the shoulder. It will also make you look shorter and older!

correcting head forward/shoulders forward

You can correct head forward/shoulders forward by stretching the pectoral muscles (chest). This version of Yoga Mudra Pose shown on the next page will target these muscles. Consistent stretching of the pectoral muscles combined with consistent strengthening of the rhomboids starts to bring head forward/shoulder forward into balance.

To strengthen the rhomboids, gently squeeze your shoulder blades together and hold for one minute. Do this exercise three to five times a day. As you squeeze your shoulder blades together to strengthen the rhomboids, your pectoral muscles are being stretched at the same time.

Everyone should stretch their chest and strengthen their rhomboids every day. It helps ensure that you have good posture for your entire life. With consistent practice it may take three to five months to retrain the muscles and correct head forward/shoulder forward. That is a pretty short time compared to how long it took you to get there!

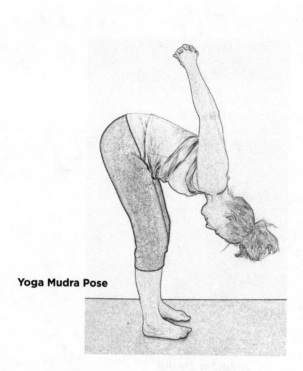

Yoga Mudra Pose

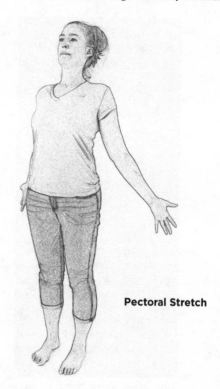

Pectoral Stretch

head tilted to the side/elevated shoulder

Head tilted to the side/elevated shoulder occurs when the scalene muscles on the side of the neck become too short on one side, thus pulling the scalene muscles on the other side into an overstretched long condition, and/or the levator scapula muscle is short on one side. This condition is often caused by improper sitting and computer positions. You may experience neck pain, chest pain, and even arm and hand pain if it impinges a nerve.

correcting head tilted to the side/elevated shoulder

You can correct head tilted to the side/elevated shoulder by stretching the scalene muscles on the side of the neck. The version of Mountain Pose shown on the next page will target this muscle. Stretch these muscles three times a day for thirty seconds.

It will also be helpful to strengthen the levator scapula muscle, which runs from the corner of the shoulder blade up into the neck. To strengthen the levator scapula, practice doing shoulder shrugs. Gently move the shoulders up toward the ears and hold for three seconds. Do this ten times. Practice this exercise different times throughout the day.

Consistent stretching of the scalenes combined with consistent strengthening of the levator scapula starts to bring head tilted/elevated shoulder back into balance. It may take three to five months to achieve lasting results.

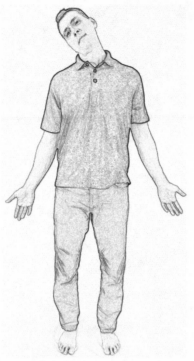 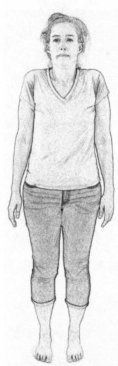

Mountain Pose head to side   **Shoulder Shrugs**

Following is a quick summary of the poses to perform to correct the five major imbalances. You will receive the quickest results by practicing these daily. Remember that the stretches should not hurt. If they do, you need to modify the pose. That is called wisdom. It is also called listening to your body.

Standing Crescent Moon Pose	corrects elevated pelvis
Supine Twist Pose	corrects rotated pelvis
Pigeon Pose	corrects a forward tilted pelvis
Bridge Pose (block between knees)	strengthens back side of body and inner thighs
Yoga Mudra Pose	corrects head forward/shoulders forward
Mountain Pose	corrects head tilted to the side/elevated shoulder

Note: If your body is not ready to practice the poses listed here to correct the five major imbalances, see chapter 13 Yoga off the Mat. I will show you modified stretches that you can do anywhere to start to correct these imbalances. The poses in this book can all be modified to a chair yoga practice.

In the next few chapters, you will learn about common symptoms and conditions caused by muscle imbalances and how to choose the correct postures to correct those conditions. Each pose will start to become easy, your hips will start to open, and your hamstrings will loosen.

Key Points

- **Eliminating the cause,** not just the symptom, is important.

- **Focus mainly on stretching muscles that are too short.**

- **Muscles will do exactly what you train them to do.**

- **The key to muscular skeletal balance is first to align the pelvis.**

- **There are three predominate pelvic imbalances**—elevated pelvis, rotated pelvis, and tilted pelvis. Many people present with all three pelvic imbalances in varying degrees.

- **There are two predominate upper body imbalances**—head forward/shoulders forward, and head tilted to the side/elevated shoulder. Many people present with both upper body imbalances in varying degrees.

- **Many people will present with all five imbalances.**

- **The five major imbalances can be corrected** in as little as three to five months with consistent practice.

- **The poses in this book can all be modified to a chair yoga practice.**

common symptoms and conditions caused by muscle imbalances—lower body

"Yoga aims to remove the root cause of all diseases, not to treat its symptoms as medical science generally attempts to do."
—Swami Vishnu-devananda

As I discussed in chapter 3, yoga was originally a spiritual system designed to help one find Ultimate Truth. The eight limbs gave guidance on how to accomplish this goal. From a larger viewpoint, yoga was intended to quiet the mind and learn to sit comfortably in meditation that would then lead to Self and God Realization.

If you have tried to meditate, you know it is a discipline that requires sustained practice and dedication. Practicing meditation becomes increasingly difficult if you are in physical pain. When physical pain keeps you from meditating, it's obviously affecting your whole life—both your body and your mood. Correcting those neuromuscular conditions stemming from muscle imbalances becomes important on a whole new level.

In my first book, ***Live Pain-free without Drugs or Surgery,*** I described the protocols I use to treat eleven common conditions:

- Tension-type headaches and migraines
- Temporomandibular joint disorder (TMJD)
- Cervical muscle strain (neck pain)
- Thoracic outlet syndrome (TOS)

- Epicondylitis, lateral or medial (tennis or golfer's elbow)

- Carpal tunnel syndrome (CTS)

- Lumbar muscle strain (low back pain)

- Piriformis syndrome (sciatica)

- Medial meniscus injury (knee pain)

- Plantar fasciitis (heel spur)

- Fibromyalgia

In this chapter you will find descriptions of prominent lower body conditions to aid you in understanding the mechanics of the condition causing your pain.

You will also find a list of common causes for each of these conditions. For the body to feel better, one must not only reduce or eliminate the pain but also remove the cause. This process often involves performing your daily activities in a slightly different way that stops the pain from returning. The old saying, "If you do what you always did, you get what you always got" applies here.

In the next chapter, I will give you a list of yoga poses that will help correct the muscle imbalances associated with the various conditions of the lower body, as well as a list of poses to avoid if you have one of these conditions. Choosing the correct poses for your condition will bring superior results.

lumbar muscle strain: low back pain

The lower back is a broad area that connects the upper body to the lower body. The pain felt in the lower back is usually caused by muscle imbalances in the lumbar and hip flexor region. The tight muscles are either too long or too short and are pulling or compressing other structures in this area, leading to pain. Tight muscles will often pull the pelvis out of alignment and/or cause the spine to be crooked and/or aggravate a disc problem. Pain may also radiate from other areas like the mid or upper back.

Low back pain is the most common complaint I hear about when I am doing individual treatments. Almost everyone will experience low back pain at some time in his or her life.

common causes of low back pain

One of the most common causes of these muscle imbalances is simply poor posture and/or improper ergonomics. Slumping at your desk or in your car rounds out the lower back. This puts considerable strain on your low back, which will likely pull the pelvis out of alignment. Keeping your back rounded for extended periods of time in your chair is a significant contributing factor in low back pain. I believe that half the back pain in the country could be eliminated if everyone sat with the proper support. By correcting your computer and driving positions, you will straighten out your back, giving yourself good posture. Your bones (the spinal column) will come back into alignment, which will help take the strain off the muscles. I will show you correct sitting, driving, and computer positions in chapter 13.

Many lifestyle habits can contribute to low back pain. The following are some of the most common I have come across in my practice:

- Long periods of improper standing
- Long periods of improper sitting
- Playing sports—especially one-sided sports like tennis and golf
- Lifting heavy objects
- Performing the wrong yoga or Pilates exercise for your current condition
- Training your muscles out of balance

These activities can all cause muscle imbalances in the low back (lumbar region), which can lead to low back pain. Limiting these activities when you have lumbar muscle strain will speed up the recovery process. An exaggerated curve in the low back, which leads to back pain, is often a sign that you are overstretching your hamstrings and not stretching your hip flexors enough.

piriformis syndrome: sciatica

The sciatic nerve has several branches coming out of the spinal cord into the lower back. Parts of the nerve run through the buttocks and down the back of each leg to the ankle and foot. A sciatic nerve irritated or compressed by a disc or a tight muscle could cause pain in the low back, buttocks, or down the leg into the foot. This is generally called sciatica. When the piriformis muscle causes this compression, it is called piriformis syndrome.

Piriformis syndrome and muscle-related sciatica are caused by muscle imbalances in the hip and buttock muscles.

common causes of sciatica

Many lifestyle habits can contribute to sciatica. The following are some of the most common I have come across in my practice.

- Biking
- Sitting improperly
- Driving, especially with a clutch

These activities can all cause muscle imbalances in the low back (lumbar region), which can lead to sciatica. Limiting these activities when you have sciatica will speed up the recovery process.

These two physiological changes can also cause sciatica:

• Spinal stenosis

• Pregnancy

knee pain and medial meniscus

The medial meniscus is a band of cartilage on the inside of the knee at the head of the tibia. Another band lies on the outside of the knee. It is a common site of injury, especially in sports. The medial meniscus acts as a shock absorber between the tibia and the femur. Large tears to the meniscus may require surgery. Small tears will respond well to the protocols in this book. The meniscus is often damaged due to muscle imbalances in the hip and leg muscles. The tight muscles are either too long or too short and pull or compress the meniscus and other structures in the knee area, leading to pain.

Knee replacements have almost doubled in the last ten years. The truth is that your knees should last longer than you do, and they will last a lot longer if the pelvis is straight, unless you have an underlying problem like rheumatoid arthritis. Think of your car. If the front end of your vehicle is out of alignment, your tires will wear out quickly. In this case, your tires are your knees. Keep the pelvis straight to save your knees. A straight pelvis will allow your knees to take the strain on them the way nature intended, and they will last you a long time.

common causes of knee pain

Many lifestyle habits can contribute to knee pain. The following are some of the most common I have come across in my practice.

• Sports

• Dancing

• Driving

• Yoga

• Weightlifting

These activities can all cause muscle imbalances around the knee, which can lead to knee or medial meniscus pain. Limiting these activities when you have knee pain will speed up the recovery process.

plantar fasciitis: heel spur

Plantar fasciitis is inflammation of the plantar fascia. This is the tissue that forms the arch of the foot. Plantar means the bottom of the foot. Fascia is connective tissue, and -itis means inflammation. A heel spur is a hook of bone that can form on the heel. Plantar fasciitis is often accompanied by a heel spur that is visible on an X-ray. Heel spurs are soft, bendable deposits of calcium that are a result of mechanical tension and inflammation. Heel spurs do not cause pain. They are an indication that plantar fasciitis may be present, which is what is causing the pain.

This condition is often due to muscle imbalances in the pelvis, lower leg, and foot muscles.

common causes of plantar fasciitis

Many lifestyle habits can contribute to plantar fasciitis. The following are some of the most common I have come across in my practice.

- Extended periods of time standing or walking
- Running
- Dancing
- Wearing improper shoes

These activities or habits can all cause muscle imbalances in the calf and foot, which can lead to plantar fasciitis. Limiting these activities when you have plantar fasciitis will speed up the recovery process. Wearing shoes that have good arch supports will help with plantar fasciitis.

fibromyalgia

Fibromyalgia means pain in the muscles, ligaments, and tendons—the soft tissues in the body. Fibromyalgia is a chronic condition with widespread pain in the muscles, ligaments, and tendons, as well as fatigue and multiple tender points. Tender points can be found in the back of the neck, shoulders, chest, lower back, hips, elbows, and knees. The pain may spread from these areas. These tender points will be on both the left and right side of the body, and both above and below the waist.

This condition is due to muscle imbalances in many different regions all over the body.

common contributors of fibromyalgia

Besides muscle imbalances, other contributors for this condition include poor dietary habits, low water intake, and a sedentary lifestyle.

People with fibromyalgia tend to wake up with body aches and stiffness. This is often because they have not had any water all night. Fibromyalgia is more common in women than in men. Other names for this condition are fibrositis, chronic muscle pain syndrome, and tension myalgias.

Fibromyalgia has no clear cause, but the following are significant contributors:

- Postural deviations
- Improper sitting posture
- Improper driving positions
- Improper computer positions

These activities can all cause muscle imbalances in the body, which can lead to fibromyalgia. Limiting or correcting these activities will speed up the recovery process.

The following habits lead to chemical imbalances in the body, muscle pain, and fatigue.

• Lack of water

• Too much caffeine

• Poor diet

The following series of yoga poses in the next chapter will help bring the pelvis back into alignment by correcting the three major hip imbalances. The focus will be on stretching the hip flexors and the hip abductor muscles. We spend far too much time in yoga stretching our hip extensors (hamstrings) and not enough on our hip flexors. We spend far too much time in yoga practicing hip openers (adductor stretch) and not enough time stretching our hip abductors. Bringing the pelvis into balance will help with all lower body conditions.

yoga sequence for the lower body

the sequence of poses I am listing can and should be modified for your particular body. Rereading chapter 5 will teach you how to stretch. Stretching properly is often more important than what you stretch. Also, feel free to substitute poses for the ones in the sequence that stretch similar muscles. Mixing up your poses from time to time is beneficial.

By practicing the poses in this chapter, you can eliminate or significantly reduce the severity of your back pain, sciatica, knee pain, plantar fasciitis, and the pain associated with fibromyalgia. These poses will start to rebalance the muscles in your body, which will give you better posture and less pain. If after practicing the poses for three to five months you still have no improvement, see your health care provider for further assessment.

note to reader:

The following series of poses are meant to be an hour and a half session. Feel free to pick and choose among the poses in the series to get started. I have given you a sample fifteen-minute practice for lower body conditions at the end of this chapter. Research has shown that you can achieve good results with a fifteen-minute practice.

Details for these poses are not provided. If you are not sure how to perform some of the poses, seek out a qualified yoga instructor to help you. These poses can all be adapted to chair yoga. The Peggy Cappy *Yoga for the Rest of Us* DVD will ease you into the world of yoga, whatever your age and ability. See http://www.peggycappy.net

yoga sequence to reduce or eliminate:
- Lumbar muscle strain (low back pain)
- Piriformis syndrome – sciatica
- Knee pain and medial meniscus
- Plantar fasciitis – heel spur
- Fibromyalgia

Asana/Mountain Pose/ Tadasana

Hold: 1–2 minutes

Comments

Chest open

Squeeze buttocks

Squeeze shoulder blades together

Pull shoulder blades down

Relax knees

Palms forward; fingers extended

Feet forward

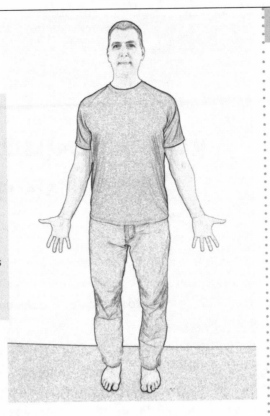

Benefits

Aligns head, shoulders, and hips

Stretches chest

Strengthens gluteal muscles and upper back

Allows for deeper breath

Pranayama

10 breaths

Comments

3-part breath; hold 3 seconds; exhale (see chapter 11)

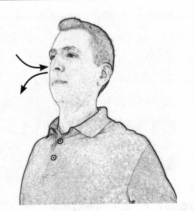

Benefits

Decreases stress

Relaxes the muscles

**Forward Bend
Backward Bend**

10–15 reps

Benefits

Increases blood flow and neural activity throughout the spine

Contributes to improved respiration, digestion, lymphatic activity, and mental clarity

Comments

Keep knees slightly bent

Do not compress low back

May keep hands on hips

**Right Side Bend
Left Side Bend**

10–15 reps

Benefits

Increases blood flow and neural activity throughout the spine

Contributes to improved respiration, digestion, lymphatic activity, and mental clarity

Comments

Keep knees slightly bent

May keep hands on hips

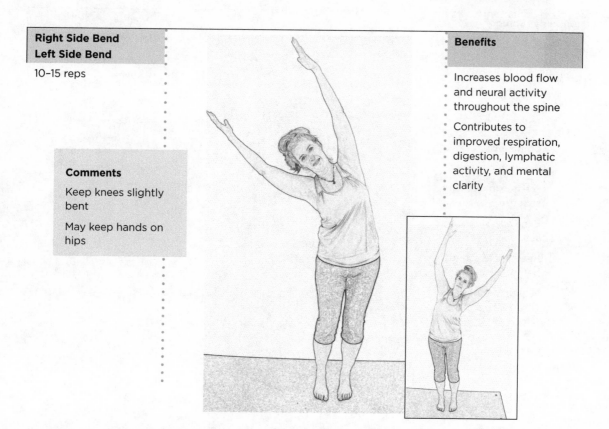

Right Spinal Twist
Left Spinal Twist

10–15 reps

Comments

Keep knees slightly bent

May keep hands on hips

May lift foot

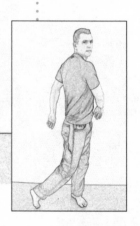

Benefits

Increases blood flow and neural activity throughout the spine

Contributes to improved respiration, digestion, lymphatic activity, and mental clarity

Shoulder Shrugs

10–15 reps

Comments

Squeeze gently

Breathe in on the squeeze

Exhale as shoulders sink down

Keep knees slightly bent

May be performed sitting

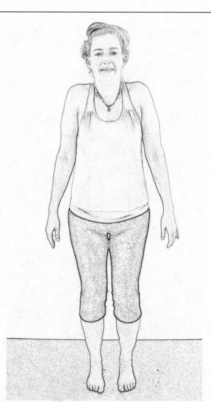

Benefits

Releases neck tension

Increases blood flow to the area

Shoulder Rolls

10–15 reps

Benefits

Lubricates shoulder joint

Brings shoulders into neutral position

Comments

Backward only

Keep knees slightly bent

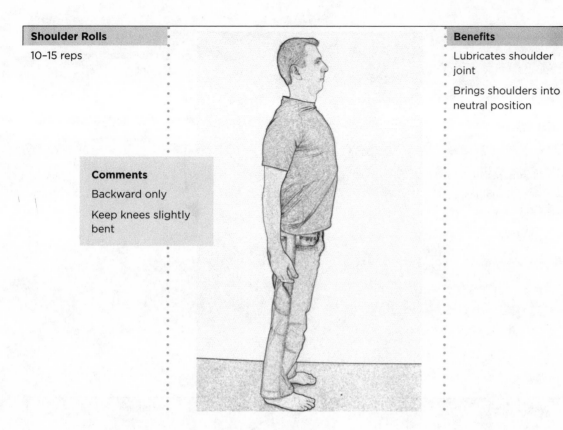

Wrist Movements

10–15 reps

Benefits

Lubricates wrist joint

Comments

Move wrists in many directions

Keep knees slightly bent

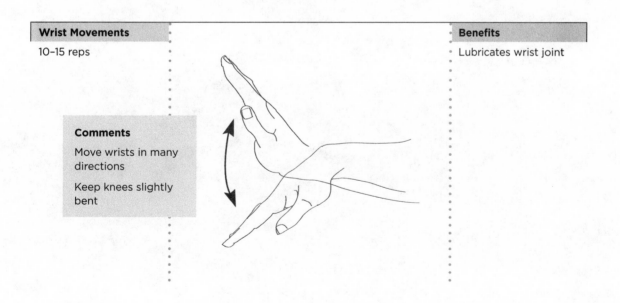

Ankle Movements

10–15 reps

Benefits

Lubricates the ankle joint

Comments

Move ankles in many directions

May leave foot on floor

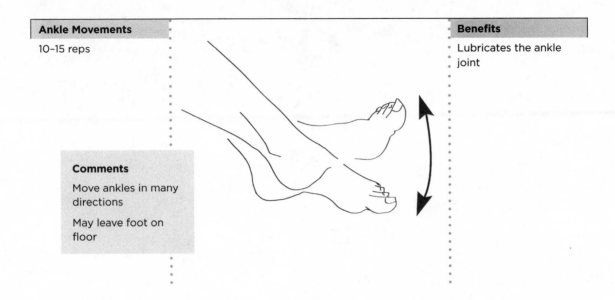

Pranayama

10 breaths

Benefits

Decreases stress

Relaxes the muscles

Comments

3-part breath; hold 3 seconds; exhale (see chapter 11)

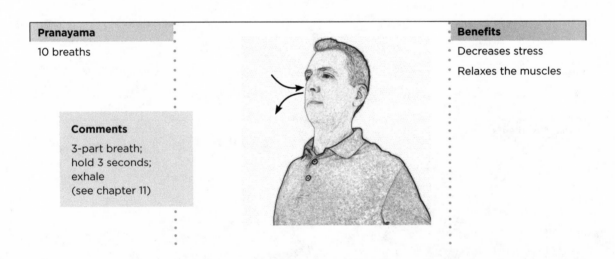

Asana Sequence: Standing Back Arch

Hold: 1–2 minutes

Comments

Stand tall; do not compress low back

Squeeze shoulder blades together and down

Keep knees slightly bent

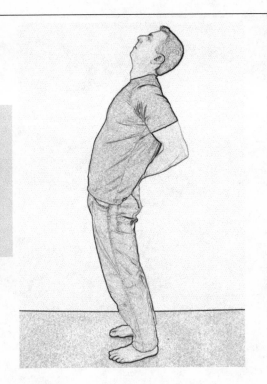

Benefits

Gently stretches chest and psoas

Strengthens the upper back

Helps with back and neck pain

Open-Hearted Warrior / Virabhadra's Pose

Hold: 1–2 minutes

Comments

Chest open/squeeze shoulder blades together

Pull shoulder blades down

Feet forward/press heel on back leg to the floor

May keep hands on hips

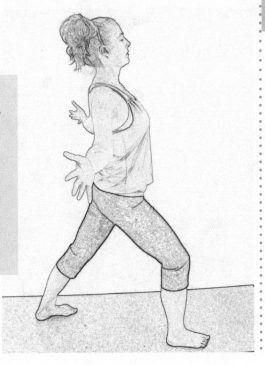

Benefits

Gently releases/stretches hip flexors

Helps to restore anterior/posterior pelvic balance

Stretches the psoas, quads, calf, and chest

Strengthens upper back

Dancer Pose / Natarajasana

Hold: 1–2 minutes

Comments

Do not stretch too deeply

Do not compress low back

Modify in the beginning if too difficult

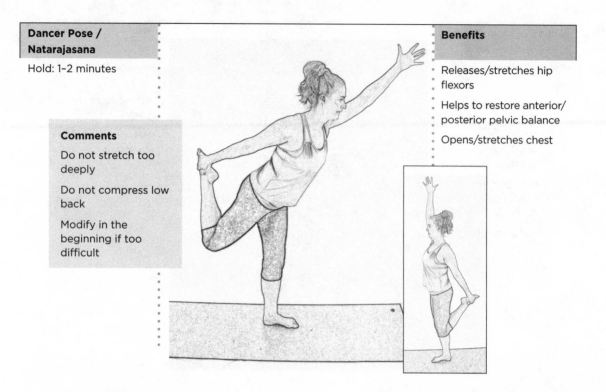

Benefits

Releases/stretches hip flexors

Helps to restore anterior/posterior pelvic balance

Opens/stretches chest

Crescent Moon Pose / Ardha Chandrasana

Hold: 1–2 minutes

Comments

May keep hands on hips

May rest arm on top of head

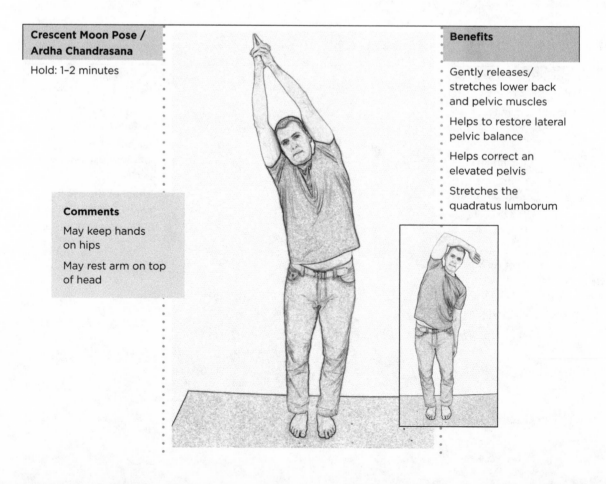

Benefits

Gently releases/stretches lower back and pelvic muscles

Helps to restore lateral pelvic balance

Helps correct an elevated pelvis

Stretches the quadratus lumborum

Crescent Moon Pose / Leg Behind

Hold: 1–2 minutes

Comments

May keep hands on hips

May rest arm on top of head

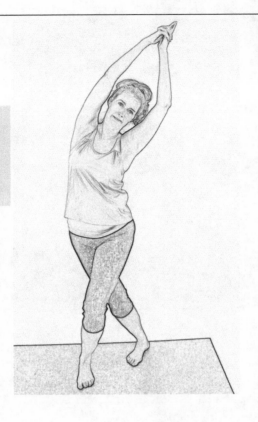

Benefits

Gently releases/stretches lower back and pelvic muscles

Helps to restore lateral pelvic balance

Stretches the quadratus lumborum and hip abductors

Hero Pose / Virasana

Hold: 1–2 minutes

Comments

Prop pillow under buttocks and/or ankles if you have knee or ankle pain

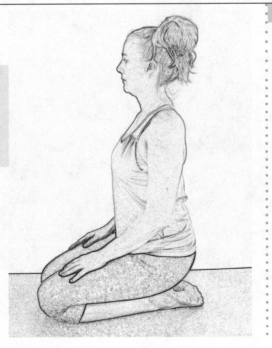

Benefits

Stretches the quads and ankles

Helps to restore anterior/posterior pelvic balance

Seated Heart Opener

Hold: 1–2 minutes

Comments

Do not strain neck

Fingers pointing away from body/squeeze shoulder blades together

May use blocks under buttocks

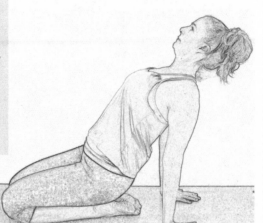

Benefits

Stretches quads, psoas, chest, and wrist flexors

Helps to restore anterior/posterior pelvic balance

Camel Pose / Ustrasana

Hold: 1–2 minutes

Comments

Start with hands on hips

Lengthen back

Squeeze buttocks

Do not compress low back

Modify in the beginning

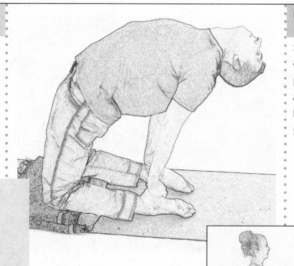

Benefits

Stretches quads, psoas, and chest

Helps to restore anterior/posterior pelvic balance

Strengthens gluteals

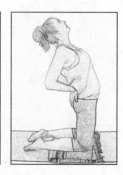

Open-Hearted Pigeon / Kapotasana

Hold: 1–2 minutes

Comments

Legs under hips

Start in lying position and work your way up

This is the antidote to sitting

Benefits

Releases hip flexors

Stretches quads, psoas, and chest

Strengthens upper back

Helps to restore anterior/posterior pelvic balance

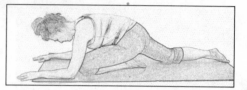

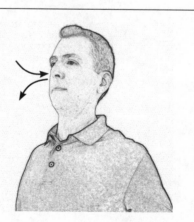

Pranayama

10 breaths

Comments

3-part breath; hold 3 seconds; exhale (see chapter 11)

Benefits

Decreases stress

Relaxes the muscles

Seated Spinal Twist / Ardha Matsyendrasana

Hold: 1–2 minutes

Comments

Improves joint alignment through greater muscle balance

Reduces ankle, knee, and hip stresses

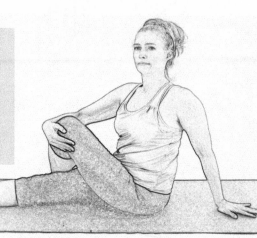

Benefits

Gently releases/relaxes hip abductors, external rotator muscles, and connective tissues of the hip and legs

Helps diminish external leg rotation

Supine Twist / Supta Matsyendrasana

Hold: 1–2 minutes

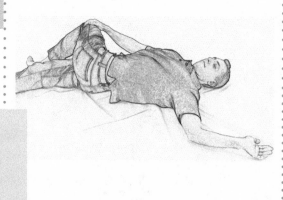

Comments

Improves joint alignment through greater muscle balance

Reduces ankle, knee, and hip stresses

Benefits

Gently releases/relaxes hip abductors, external rotator muscles, and connective tissues of the hip and legs

Helps diminish external leg rotation

Cow Face Pose / Gomukhasana

Hold: 1–2 minutes

Comments

Modify on back

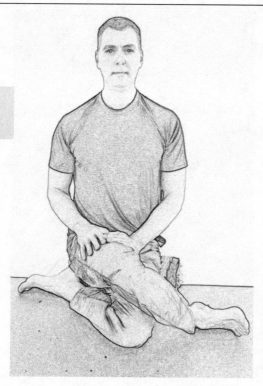

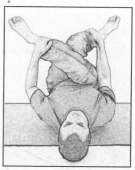

Benefits

Releases/relaxes hip abductors, external rotator muscles, and connective tissues of the hip and legs

Helps diminish external leg rotation

Sphinx Pose / Salamba Bhujangasana

Hold: 1–2 minutes

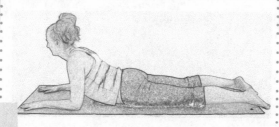

Comments

Squeeze shoulder blades together

Squeeze buttocks

Do not strain neck or lower back

Benefits

Stretches psoas and chest

Strengthens upper back

Helps to restore anterior/posterior pelvic balance

Pranayama

10 breaths

Comments

3-part breath;
hold 3 seconds;
exhale
(see chapter 11)

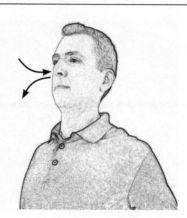

Benefits

- Decreases stress
- Relaxes the muscles

**Bridge Pose / Setu
Bandha Sarvangasana**

Hold: 1–2 minutes

Comments

Place block between
knees to strengthen
the adductors

Squeeze shoulder
blades together

Squeeze buttocks

May keep arms
alongside of body

Press arms into mat

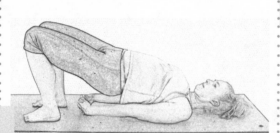

Benefits

- Strengthens gluteal
  muscles, hamstrings,
  and rhomboids
- Diminishes anterior
  pelvic tilt
- Great for back pain

Upward Facing Dog / Urdhva Mukha Svanasana

Hold: 1–2 minutes

Comments

Squeeze shoulder blades together and down

Squeeze buttocks

Do not strain neck or lower back

Lift thighs off mat

May substitute cobra pose

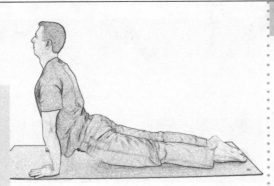

Benefits

Strengthens upper and lower back muscles

Stretches chest, psoas, and quads

Helps to restore anterior/posterior pelvic balance

Child's Pose / Balasana

Hold: 1–2 minutes

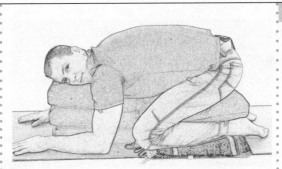

Benefits

Stretches the quads, ankles, and low back

Takes the strain off the psoas

Great for low back pain

Comments

Prop pillow under the buttocks and/or ankles if you have knee or ankle pain

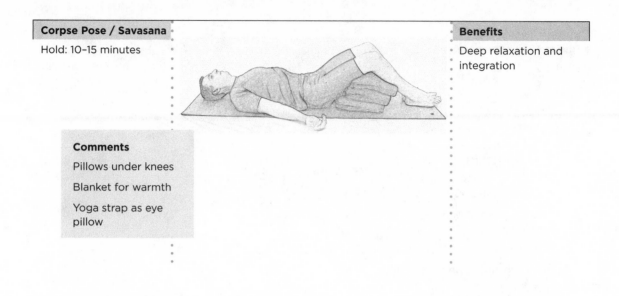

Corpse Pose / Savasana

Hold: 10–15 minutes

Benefits

Deep relaxation and integration

Comments

Pillows under knees

Blanket for warmth

Yoga strap as eye pillow

poses that aggravate lower body conditions

Practicing the above poses will generally start to bring the body into balance. However, additionally practicing the following poses could take much longer to bring the muscles into balance. The poses listed below are stretching muscles that are typically too long already. Stretching these muscles may slow your progress.

- Downward Facing Dog – Adho Mukha Svanasana
- Seated Forward Bend – Paschimottanasana
- Wide-Legged Seated Forward Bend – Upavistha Konasana
- Hamstring Stretches
- Adductor Stretches
- Bound Angle – Baddha Konasana
- Easy Pose – Sukhasana
- Lotus Pose – Padmasana
- Frog Pose – Mandukasana
- Triangle Pose – Trikonasana
- Tree Pose - Vrksasana

These poses can be brought back into your practice once your symptoms start to alleviate.

15-minute sequence for lower body conditions

Here is a sequence of poses to practice if you have a busy schedule and don't have time for the full practice or if you have not yet built up the endurance for the full practice. Remember, don't force your body where it doesn't want to go yet. It will slowly open up with consistent practice. This sequence of poses, which I have taken from the above flow, will take you 10–15 minutes. Once in the morning and once in the evening has proven to bring great benefits.

- Mountain Pose (Tadasana)
- Six Movements of the Spine:
- Forward Bend / Backward Bend
- Left Side Bend / Right Side Bend
- Left Spinal Twist / Right Spinal Twist
- Shoulder Rolls
- Open Hearted Warrior / Virabhadra's Pose
- Seated Heart Opener
- Bridge Pose / Setu Bandha Sarvangasana
- Supine Twist / Supta Matsyendrasana
- Open Hearted Pigeon / Kapotasana

After you have practiced for a month, begin to substitute some of the poses in the longer sequence for those in the shorter one. You will receive greater benefit by varying the poses and not always practicing the same ones. Also read chapter 13 and adapt the yoga off-the-mat practices that I am recommending. Practicing both on and off the mat will give you quicker results.

In the next chapter, we will look at common upper body conditions we can correct by wisely choosing which poses to perform.

Key Points

- **80% of the pain** we will feel in our lives is due to neuromuscular conditions stemming from muscle imbalances.
- **Five common lower body ailments** are:
  - Lumbar Muscle Strain (Low Back Pain)
  - Piriformis Syndrome – Sciatica
  - Knee Pain and Medial Meniscus Pain
  - Plantar Fasciitis – Heel Spur
  - Fibromyalgia
- **By practicing the poses** in this chapter, you can eliminate or significantly reduce the severity of your back pain, sciatic pain, knee pain, foot pain, and fibromyalgia.
- **The sequence of poses** in this chapter can and should be modified for your particular body condition. Never stretch into pain.

common symptoms and conditions

caused by muscle imbalances—upper body

"To keep the body in good health is a duty . . . otherwise, we shall not be able to keep our mind strong and clear."
—Buddha

Pain in the upper back, shoulders, head, and neck are common in the clients I treat. Most people have experienced pain in these areas at some time in their lives. Most of these uncomfortable conditions originate from improper sitting positions. Chapter 13 will teach you how to sit comfortably with no pain.

In this chapter, you will find descriptions of various conditions to aid you in understanding the mechanics of what is causing your pain. Again, all of these conditions are caused by muscle imbalances. These tight muscles pull the bones out of alignment, which can cause muscle pain, disc problems, nerve compressions, and tendonitis.

You will also find a list of common causes for each of these conditions. For the body to feel better, it is important not only to reduce or eliminate the pain but also to remove the cause. The same as with lower body pain, this process often involves doing your daily activities in a slightly different way that stops the pain from returning.

I will give you a list of yoga poses that will help correct the muscle imbalances associated with the various conditions, and also a list of poses to avoid.

tension-type headaches and migraines

The most common type of headache is a tension-type headache. These are sometimes called stress headaches. A headache is one of the most common reasons people seek medical help.

Recent research shows that most headaches are a combination of both tension and migraine. Whether a headache is caused by the muscle tension or the muscle tension results from the headache, treating that muscle tension can provide significant relief from the pain.

Tension-type headaches are often due to muscle imbalances in the neck and shoulder muscles. Even though the head is where you feel the pain, the cause is usually a strained muscle in the neck or shoulder area.

Many migraine headaches are also caused by muscle imbalances, but some are not. Other factors contributing to a migraine are diet, brain chemical imbalances, lack of water, and hormonal imbalances. This chapter addresses migraines and headaches caused by muscle imbalances. If the protocols listed in this chapter are not working, check with your healthcare provider, as you might have a headache not caused by muscle imbalances or dehydration.

common causes of headaches

Many lifestyle habits can contribute to a headache. The following are some of the most common I have come across in my practice.

- **Poor posture,** especially head forward of the body or arms held extended for long periods of time. These postures are typical of driving and computer positions. They put a lot of strain on the neck and shoulder muscles that can lead to a headache.

- **Emotional or mental stress,** anxiety, TMJ and/or teeth grinding at night. This kind of stress makes your tight muscles even tighter.

- **Fatigue and/or lack of sleep.** Fatigue upsets the chemical balance in the body and can lead to a headache.

- **Dehydration.** Lack of water can make your joints and/or muscles ache a lot more and lead to pain in the head.

- **Eyestrain.** Eyestrain can cause a headache due to muscle imbalances around the eye. If you wear glasses, make sure your prescription is up to date; if you do not wear glasses, see your eye doctor, as you might need them. Periodically give your eyes a rest. While at the computer, take a break and stare out the window for a few minutes. This shift in attention gives the eye a different focal point and helps to relieve eyestrain.

- **Caffeine withdrawal.** When giving up caffeine, always do so slowly. Slowly coming off caffeine and keeping well hydrated can mitigate the effects of withdrawal.

- **Hunger.** Low blood sugar can also lead to a headache. Eat a balanced diet at regular intervals to keep the blood sugar even. Do not skip meals. Protein and healthy fat help to keep blood sugar levels more even.

- **Reading in bed with head propped up.** This is a common practice that leads to many headaches. This position significantly strains the neck and shoulder muscles.
- **Low or high blood pressure.**

temporomandibular joint disorder – TMJ

TMJ is the common abbreviation for temporomandibular joint disorder. The temporomandibular joint, sometimes called the "jaw joint," is in front of the ear. The joint attaches the lower jaw to the skull and allows you to open and close your mouth, chew, and speak. A malfunctioning jaw joint can be very painful.

If you place two fingers on your jaw in front of the ear and chew, you can feel the joint moving. TMJ is a condition where tight muscles put pressure on the joint and, in more severe cases, even pull it out of joint.

Tight muscles, or muscle imbalances, in the neck, face, and jaw muscles often start with a crooked pelvis because the spine sits on the pelvis. If the pelvis is crooked, the spine is crooked.

An estimated ten million Americans suffer from TMJ. You can have tight, sore jaw muscles and not have TMJ. The protocol for getting rid of a tight jaw is the same as for TMJ. A tight jaw is often a precursor to TMJ.

common causes of TMJ

Many lifestyle habits can contribute to TMJ. The following are some of the most common I have come across in my practice:

- **Tight muscles around the jaw** (especially the masseter), grinding teeth, and stress. This kind of stress makes your tight muscles even tighter. Try the breathing exercise described in chapter 11.
- **Chewing gum, poor posture, reading in bed,** cradling a phone between your ear and shoulder, and playing a wind or string instrument are examples of activities that put a lot of strain on the neck, shoulder, and jaw muscles and can lead to TMJ.
- **Head-forward posture.**

cervical muscle strain (neck pain)

Neck pain can occur due to muscular tightness in both the neck and upper back that could lead to compressed nerves or disc issues in this region. A misaligned pelvis is also a contributor to neck pain. Almost everybody will experience a tight, sore neck at some point in their lifetime.

The neck or cervical spine is that part of the body that connects the head to the trunk. It is comprised of muscles, nerves, arteries, bones, and discs. These discs act as shock absorbers between the cervical vertebrae.

The pain felt in the neck is usually caused by muscle imbalances in the neck, shoulder, or upper back.

common causes of neck pain

In my twenty-five years of experience, I have worked with only a handful of people who did not have a tight neck. One of the most common causes of muscle imbalances in the neck is simply poor posture and/or improper ergonomics. Slumping at your desk or in your car pushes your head forward of your body, putting a lot of strain on your neck and shoulders, which now have to hold up your head. The average head weighs between eight and twelve pounds. If you tried to hold that much weight with your arms, you probably would not last more than five minutes. Yet we ask our neck and shoulder muscles to hold that weight all day long. These muscles are not designed to hold up your head. They are meant to move your head in different directions, not hold them in the same position for extended periods of time. By correcting your computer and driving positions, you will bring your head over your shoulders, giving yourself good posture. Your bones will be holding up your head, which will take the strain off the muscles.

Many lifestyle habits contribute to neck pain. The following are some of the most common I have come across in my practice:

- **Improper sitting positions, driving positions, standing positions, and computer positions** lead to head forward posture that can cause cervical muscle strain and perhaps lead to a disc problem.

- **Emotional stress** can also aggravate cervical muscle strain. Try the breathing exercise described in chapter 11.

- **Cradling the phone** between shoulder and ear or holding a phone to the ear may cause a muscle imbalance.

thoracic outlet syndrome (TOS)

The thoracic outlet is the space between the collarbone and the first rib. Thoracic outlet syndrome (TOS) is a compression of the nerves and/or blood vessels that affect the brachial plexus (nerves and blood vessels that pass into the arms from the neck). This compression is due to muscle imbalances in the neck, chest, back, and pelvis, if the compression is not due to the presence of an extra rib called a cervical rib. Tight muscles can lead to pain and/or tingling and numbness in the arms or hands.

common causes of thoracic outlet syndrome

Many lifestyle habits can contribute to thoracic outlet syndrome. The following are some of the most common I have come across in my practice:

- Repetitive activities that require the arms to be held over the head or outstretched
- Poor posture, especially head forward
- Improper computer and driving positions
- Cradling the phone between shoulder and ear or holding a phone to the ear
- Riding a bike
- Whiplash
- Gardening

These activities can all cause muscle imbalances in the neck, shoulders, and pelvis, which can cause compression of the brachial plexus in the thoracic outlet.

The series of yoga poses in the next chapter are designed to bring the muscles in the upper body back into balance. These poses will all help with the conditions discussed in this chapter. The focus will be on stretching the chest muscles and strengthening the upper back muscles. Remember that most people have the same muscle imbalances with some variations. Almost everyone will present with muscles that are too short in the front, especially the chest muscles. Almost everyone will present with muscles that are too long in the back, especially the rhomboids and trapezius muscles. These imbalances are mainly caused by a lifetime of sitting and all the looking down we do with our devices.

yoga sequence
for upper body

the sequence of poses in this chapter can and should be modified for your particular body. Do not try to force yourself into the full expression of the pose. Remember that this is a practice. It will take time to achieve the full expression of a pose. Rereading chapter 5 will teach you how to stretch. For extra benefit, substitute other poses for the ones in the sequence that stretch similar muscles.

By practicing the poses in this book, you can eliminate or significantly reduce the severity of your headaches, neck pain, jaw pain, and the pain associated with thoracic outlet syndrome (pain & tingling in the arms and hands). These poses will start to rebalance the muscles in your body, which will give you better posture and less pain. Your chest will open up, your shoulders will not round forward anymore, and your head will come back over your body. You will look younger! If, after practicing the poses for three to five months, you still have no improvement, see your health care provider for further assessment.

note to reader:

The following series of poses are meant to be an hour and a half session. Feel free to pick some of the poses in the series to get started. I have given you a sample fifteen-minute sequence for upper body conditions at the end of this chapter. Practicing for fifteen minutes is better than no practice at all.

Details for these poses are not provided. If you are not sure how to perform some of the poses, seek out a qualified yoga instructor to help you. These poses can all be adapted to chair yoga. If you opt for chair yoga, The Peggy Cappy Yoga for the Rest of Us DVD will ease you into the world of yoga, whatever your age and ability. See http://www.peggycappy.net

yoga poses to reduce or eliminate:

- Tension-type headaches and migraines
- Temporomandibular joint disorder (TMJD)
- Cervical muscle strain (neck pain)
- Thoracic outlet syndrome

warmups

Mountain Pose / Tadasana
Hold: 1–2 minutes

Comments

Chest open

Squeeze buttocks

Squeeze shoulder blades together

Pull shoulder blades down

Relax knees

Palms forward; fingers extended

Feet forward

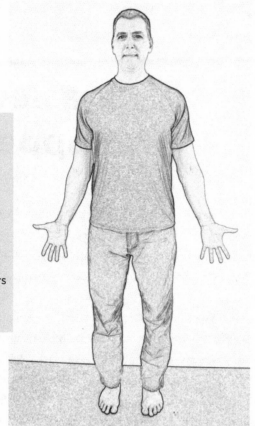

Benefits
Aligns head, shoulders, and hips

Stretches chest

Strengthens gluteal muscles and upper back

Allows for deeper breath

Pranayama
10 breaths

Comments

3-part breath; hold 3 seconds; exhale (see chapter 11)

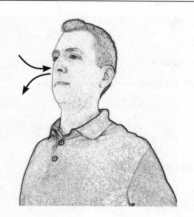

Benefits
Decreases stress

Relaxes the muscles

Forward Bend / Backward Bend

10–15 reps

Comments

Keep knees slightly bent

Do not compress low back

May keep hands on hips

Benefits

Increases blood flow and neural activity throughout the spine

Contributes to improved respiration, digestion, lymphatic activity, and mental clarity

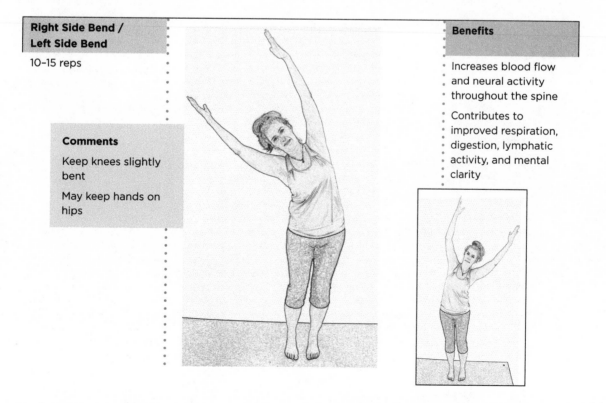

Right Side Bend / Left Side Bend

10–15 reps

Comments

Keep knees slightly bent

May keep hands on hips

Benefits

Increases blood flow and neural activity throughout the spine

Contributes to improved respiration, digestion, lymphatic activity, and mental clarity

Right Spinal Twist / Left Spinal Twist

10–15 reps

Comments

Keep knees slightly bent

May keep hands on hips

May lift foot

Benefits

Increases blood flow and neural activity throughout the spine

Contributes to improved respiration, digestion, lymphatic activity, and mental clarity

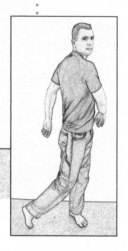

Shoulder Shrugs

10–15 reps

Comments

Squeeze gently

Breathe in on the squeeze

Exhale as shoulders sink down

Keep knees slightly bent

Can be done seated

Benefits

Releases neck tension

Increases blood flow to the area

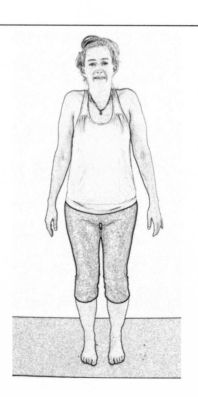

Shoulder Rolls

10–15 reps

Comments

Backward only

Keep knees slightly bent

Benefits

Lubricates shoulder joint

Brings shoulders into neutral position

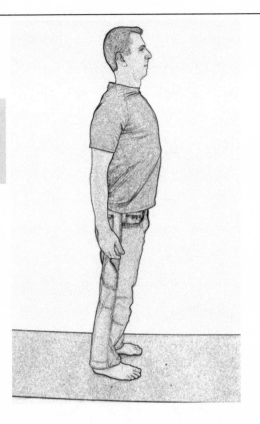

Wrist Movements

10–15 reps

Comments

Move wrists in many directions

Keep knees slightly bent

Benefits

Lubricates wrist joint

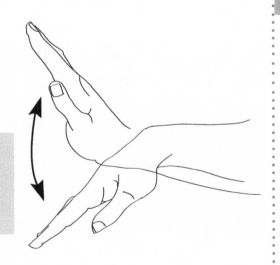

Ankle Movements		Benefits
10–15 reps		Lubricates the ankle joint

Comments

Move ankles in many directions

May leave foot on floor

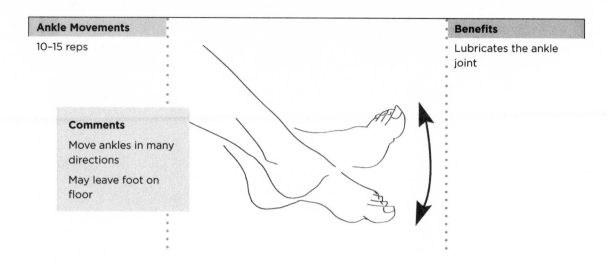

Pranayama		Benefits
10 breaths		Decreases stress
		Relaxes the muscles

Comments

3-part breath; hold 3 seconds; exhale

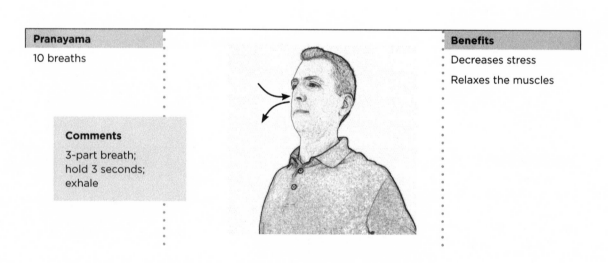

Posterior Neck Stretch

Using Contract/Relax

Comments

Pull head forward until you feel a slight stretch

Gently push backward into your hands for 5 or 6 seconds

Pull head forward into a deeper stretch

Repeat as necessary

This will stretch the muscles on the back of your neck

Do not stretch too deeply as this is often overstretched

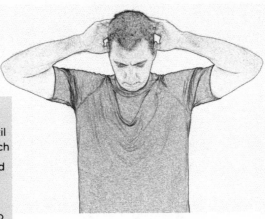

Benefits

Increases muscle and joint range of motion of the cervical spine

Lateral Neck Stretch

Using Contract/Relax

Comments

Pull head to one side until you feel a slight stretch

Gently push back into your hand for 5 or 6 seconds

Pull head to side into a deeper stretch

Repeat as necessary

Repeat on other side

This will stretch the muscles on the side of your neck

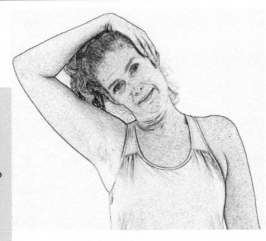

Benefits

Increases muscle and joint range of motion of the cervical spine

Anterior Neck Stretch

Using Contract/Relax

Comments

Rotate head to one side until you feel a slight stretch

Gently rotate back into your hand for 5 or 6 seconds

Rotate head to side into a deeper stretch

Repeat as necessary

Repeat on other side

This will stretch the muscles on the front of your neck

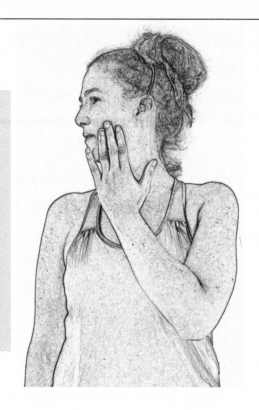

Benefits

Increases muscle and joint range of motion of the cervical spine

Asana Sequence: Standing Back Arch

Hold: 1–2 minutes

Comments

Stand tall

Do not compress low back

Squeeze shoulder blades together

Keep knees slightly bent

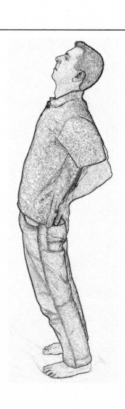

Benefits

Gently stretches chest and psoas

Strengthens the upper back

Helps with back and neck pain

Trains head to come back over shoulders

Chest Opener

Hold: 1–2 minutes

Benefits

Gently releases/ stretches chest

Strengthens the upper back

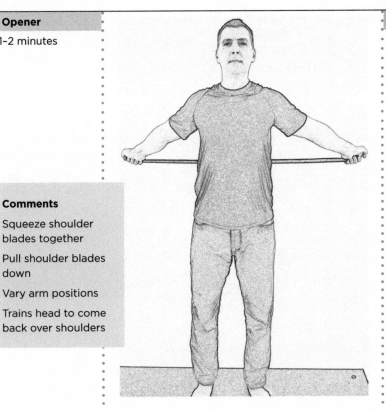

Comments

Squeeze shoulder blades together

Pull shoulder blades down

Vary arm positions

Trains head to come back over shoulders

Yoga Mudra

Hold: 1–2 minutes

Benefits

Stretches chest and low back

Strengthens upper back

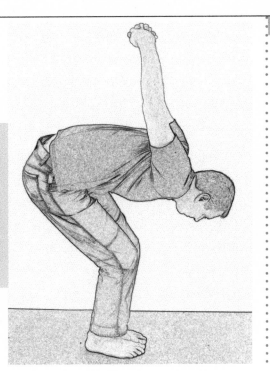

Comments

Feet slightly apart

Keep knees bent

Bend at the hip

Squeeze shoulder blades together

Trains head to come back over shoulders

Open Hearted Warrior/ Virabhadra's Pose

Hold: 1–2 minutes

Comments

Chest open/squeeze shoulder blades to-gether

Pull shoulder blades down

Feet forward/press heel on back leg to the floor

May keep hands on hips

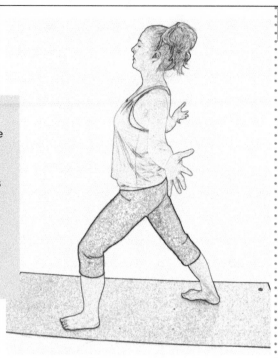

Benefits

Gently releases/ stretches hip flexors

Helps to restore anterior/posterior pelvic balance

Stretches the psoas, quads, calf, and chest

Strengthens upper back

Trains head to come back over shoulders

Pranayama

10 breaths

Comments

3-part breath; hold 3 seconds; exhale

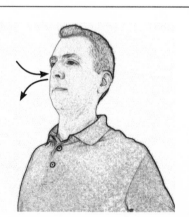

Benefits

Decreases stress

Relaxes the muscles

Cat/Cow

Hold: 5-10 Reps

Benefits

Increases function and ROM of lumbar/sacral spine, SI, and hip joints

Stretches chest and low back

Stretches forearm flexors

Comments

Do not strain lower back

Don't perform if this causes back pain

Use blocks to keep wrists straight if you have wrist pain

May place folded blanket under knees

May be done in a standing position

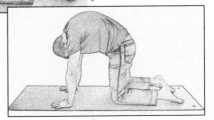

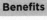

Melting Heart Pose

Hold: 1-2 minutes

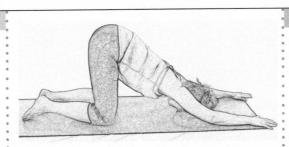

Benefits

Stretches chest, spine, and shoulders

Comments

Do not put strain on neck

Head rests on floor or cushion

Hips directly over knees

May use bolster under chest/blanket under knees

Child's Pose / Balasana

Hold: 1–2 minutes

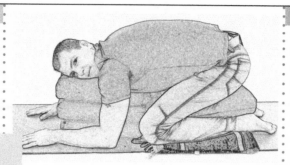

Benefits

Stretches the quads, ankles, and low back

Takes strain off the psoas

Great for low back pain

Comments

Prop pillow under buttocks and/or ankles if you have knee or ankle pain

Open Hearted Pigeon / Kapotasana

Hold: 1–2 minutes

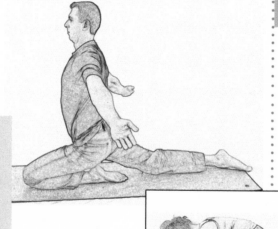

Benefits

IReleases hip flexors

Stretches quads, psoas, and chest

Strengthens upper back

Trains head to come back over shoulders

Comments

Legs under hips

Start in lying position and work your way up

The antidote to sitting

Sphinx Pose/ Salamba Bhujangasana

Hold: 1–2 minutes

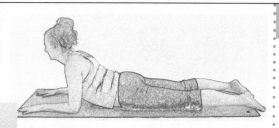

Comments

Squeeze shoulder blades together

Squeeze buttocks

Do not strain neck or lower back

Benefits

Stretches psoas and chest

Strengthens upper back

Trains head to come back over shoulders

Camel Pose/Ustrasana

Hold: 1–2 minutes

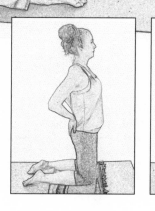

Comments

Start with hands on hips

Lengthen back

Squeeze buttocks

Do not compress low back

Modify in the beginning

Benefits

Stretches quads, psoas, and chest

Helps to restore anterior/posterior pelvic balance

Trains head to come back over shoulders

Strengthens gluteals

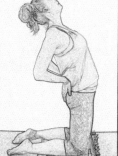

Child's Pose/ Balasana

Hold: 1–2 minutes

Comments

Prop pillow under buttocks and/or ankles if you have knee or ankle pain

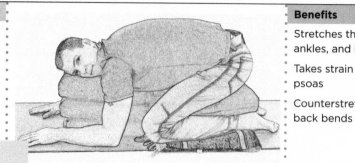

Benefits

Stretches the quads, ankles, and low back

Takes strain off the psoas

Counterstretch for back bends

Upward Facing Dog / Urdhva Mukha Svanasana

Hold: 1–2 minutes

Comments

Squeeze shoulder blades together and down

Squeeze buttocks together

Do not strain neck or lower back

Lift thighs off mat

May substitute cobra pose

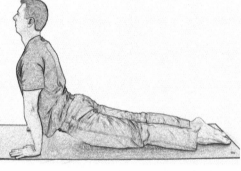

Benefits

Strengthens upper and lower back muscles

Stretches chest, psoas, and quads

Trains head to come back over shoulders

Knees to Chest Pose / Apanasana

Hold: 1–2 minutes

Comments

Alternative to child's pose

May do one leg at a time

Keep back flat on mat

Counterpose for back bends

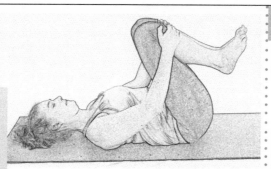

Benefits

Stretches low back

Bridge Pose / Setu Bandha Sarvangasana

Hold: 1–2 minutes

Comments

Place block between knees to strengthen the adductors

Squeeze shoulder blades together

Squeeze buttocks

May keep arms alongside of body

Press arms into mat

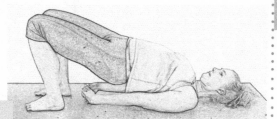

Benefits

Strengthens gluteal muscles, hamstrings, and rhomboids

Diminishes anterior pelvic tilt

Great for back pain

Supported Fish

1–2 minutes

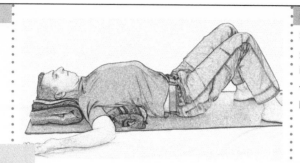

Benefits

Stretches the chest

Stretches the intercostal muscles

Trains head to come back over shoulders

Comments

Prop so as not to strain neck

Keep palms up

Breathe deeply and slowly from the belly

Corpse Pose / Savasana

Hold: 10–15 minutes

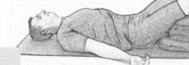

Benefits

Deep relaxation and integration

Comments

Pillows under knees

Blanket for warmth

Yoga strap as eye pillow

poses that aggravate upper body conditions

Practicing the above poses will generally bring the upper body into balance. However, additionally practicing the following poses could take much longer to bring the muscles into balance. The poses listed below are stretching muscles that are typically too long already and may slow your progress.

Remember that muscles that are too long and tight hurt more than those that are too short; it often feels good to stretch them, but that will only hinder your progress.

Eagle arms

Plank

Seated Forward Fold – Paschimottanasana

Boat – Navasana

Warrior poses with arms behind

Headstand – Sirsasana

Shoulder stand – Salamba Sarvangasana

Plow – Sarvandasana

These poses can be brought back into your routine once your symptoms start to alleviate and your body comes back into balance.

15-minute sequence for upper body conditions

Following is a sequence of poses to practice if you have a busy schedule and don't have time for the full practice or if you have not yet built up the endurance for the full practice. Remember, don't force your body where it doesn't want to go yet. It will slowly open up with consistent practice. This sequence of poses, which I have taken from the above flow, will take 10–15 minutes. Once in the morning and once in the evening will bring great benefits.

Mountain Pose (Tadasana)

Six Movements of the Spine:

Forward Bend / Backward Bend

Left Side Bend / Right Side Bend

Left Spinal Twist / Right Spinal Twist

Shoulder Rolls

Open Hearted Warrior / Virabhadra's Pose

Seated Heart Opener

Chest Opener

Camel Pose / Ustrasana

Sphinx Pose / Salamba Bhujangasana

Supported Fish

After you have practiced for a month, substitute some of the poses in the longer sequence for those in the shorter one. You will receive greater benefit by varying the poses and not always practicing the same ones. Also, read chapter 13 and adapt the yoga-off-the-mat practices I recommend. You will receive quicker results by practicing both on and off the mat.

In the next chapter, you will discover the many beneficial effects that proper breathing has for helping you stretch and for your overall health and well-being.

Key Points

- **About 80% of the pain we will feel** in our lives is due to neuromuscular conditions often stemming from muscle imbalances.
- **Four common upper body ailments are:**
  - Tension-type headaches and migraines
  - Temporomandibular joint disorder (TMJD)
  - Cervical muscle strain (neck pain)
  - Thoracic outlet syndrome
- **By practicing the poses in this book, you can eliminate or significantly reduce** the severity of your headaches, neck pain, jaw pain, and the pain associated with thoracic outlet syndrome (pain and tingling in the arms and hands).
- **The sequence of poses** in this chapter can and should be modified for your particular body.

breath is a powerful ally

"The breath is the key to unlocking your body's potential."
—Baron Baptiste

a discussion of yoga would not be complete without examining the benefits of breath, both as a tool for helping us stretch more deeply and more safely and as a tool for health and well-being. In yoga, this practice of breathing is called pranayama. It is one of the eight limbs of yoga mentioned in chapter 3. The ancient yogis believed that pranayama was a key practice to health and vitality. In our stressful world, pranayama is even more important today.

Pranayama is a Sanskrit word that translates to "control of the breath." I like to think of it as intentional breathing. Prana in Sanskrit means the life force, the vital energy of the body. This force is also called Chi in many eastern traditions.

Many different pranayama exercises are practiced today. Entire books have been written on this subject alone. For our purposes, we are going to focus on:

- learning to breathe with a full breath

- having the exhale longer than the inhale

- how to breathe when practicing asana to achieve the best results

Mastering these aspects of pranayama will go a long way to achieving health and well-being.

breath is life

Few people pay attention to their breath. But even though it is automatic, breathing is an important aspect of our lives. Oxygen is the most important "nutrient" you can put into your body. The way you inhale and exhale determines how much vital energy you have in your body. You can go thirty days without food and many days without water and have a chance for survival, but you cannot go more than minutes without oxygen. Clearly, oxygen is vital to all human life.

Most people are what we call "chest breathers." This means that most people are filling the upper third of their lungs with oxygen with every breath and ignoring the bottom two-thirds of their lungs. They are only taking in 30%–40% of the oxygen available to them and are not completely expelling the carbon dioxide (a waste product) in the lower part of the lungs! Breathing at 30% is enough to keep you alive, but it is not enough to thrive.

We were all born into this world with an innate ability to breathe properly. Observe how a baby breathes. They take a full, deep, slow breath with each inhale. Observe your own breath. You will likely notice that your breathing is shallow and rapid, which is common for adults. Poor posture, slouching in a chair, lack of exercise, tight clothing, multitasking, stress, and poor air quality are some of the components of modern life that lead to shallow breathing. Not breathing optimally has many adverse effects on the body and mind. We need to relearn how to take a "belly breath"— that is, to breathe to our full capacity.

Try this experiment:

Look at a clock that can count seconds. Sit in a chair and observe how many times you breathe in a minute. Most people will breathe fifteen to twenty breaths in a minute. That is too fast for optimal health. Rapid, shallow breathing has been linked to stress and anxiety. With an intentional breathing practice, you could lower that to eight to twelve breaths. Slower, deeper breathing has been linked to many health benefits that we will discuss later in this chapter. By breathing slower and deeper, you calm your nervous system and expel more toxins from the lungs.

benefits of taking a full breath

If you have been to a yoga class, you have heard the instructor say to pay attention to your breath and breathe more fully. Pranayama is a paramount practice that is not explained or emphasized well enough in many classes. The truth is the depth and rhythm of your breath directly affects the health of your body and your state of mind.

An intentional breathing practice has many benefits. Here are some of the most prominent:

calms the nervous system—reduces stress and anxiety

Many psychotherapists, yoga teachers, and stress specialists recommend slow, deep breathing as a way to reduce stress and anxiety in the body and mind. The world we live in can be stressful. We often live in a constant "fight or flight" state. Our bodies were designed for survival when danger is present. If our well-being was threatened, such as being chased by a tiger, our bodies would release adrenaline, which would make our muscles stronger and tighter. This adrenaline response would help us to run faster and/or be able to fight off that tiger. The adrenaline is then depleted after we use it, and our body goes back to its normal state.

In the modern world, many everyday occurrences can trigger the release of adrenaline in our bodies. This could be anything from the boss yelling at you at work to getting the kids ready for school to watching bad news on the TV. When adrenaline is released, your muscles tense, getting ready to "fight or flight." Our breathing becomes shallow and rapid. Since we don't fight or flight, the tension in the body remains for a much longer time than if we had taken some action by running or fighting. This condition of tight muscles due to the activation of our sympathetic nervous system is often referred to as stress. Chronic stress then turns into anxiety. This stress is the underlying cause of many illnesses in our modern life.

In many studies, slow, deep breathing for as little as ten minutes has been shown to calm the sympathetic nervous system, reduce stress and anxiety, and bring the body back into homeostasis (balance).

helps alleviate muscular pain

As we discussed in chapter 1, tight muscles lead to less oxygen in the tissues in those areas. **This lack of optimal oxygen causes much of a person's pain.** An intentional breathing practice will relax the nervous system and thus the muscles, allowing for increased blood flow to the tissues.

In my practice as a neuromuscular therapist, I have observed that deep, intentional breathing will often reduce or eliminate many types of neuromuscular pain.

increases the vital energy in the body

When we inhale, oxygen is taken into small air sacs in the lungs. This oxygen is essential for producing ATP (adenosine triphosphate), the chemical basis of energy production in the body. The body sends the oxygen to every cell; at the same time, when you exhale, carbon dioxide (a waste product of energy production) is moved out of the body. When we are able to take in more oxygen through intentional breathing, we will experience more energy and more mental clarity, and we will expel more toxins from the body. It does not take long to feel the difference in your body.

removes toxins from the body

We expel an estimated 70% of the toxins in the body through the lungs when we exhale. Urine, feces, and sweat account for the remaining 30% of waste products removed from the body. If we are not breathing optimally, our lymphatic system is greatly stressed.

The lymph system is the drainage system that helps us eliminate toxins and waste products from the body. It is often called the sewer system of the body. Toxins build up in the body due to inactivity and shallow breathing. Every cell in your body is surrounded by lymph fluid. Your body contains more lymph fluid than blood.

The lymph system, unlike the circulatory system, does not have a pump to move the waste. The lymph moves when we move our muscles. Deep belly breathing helps to speed up the movement of the lymph. Keeping the lymph moving is the best health practice for a vital, disease-free life. One of the best ways to keep your lymph moving adequately is by a daily practice of brisk walking, swinging your arms at the same time, and a daily practice of deep breathing.

fun fact: *Other than shallow breathing, another reason we do not get enough oxygen is that the air we breathe today contains less oxygen than it once did. When scientists measure the percentage of oxygen in the air in a pristine environment such as a country setting with lots of trees and few cars, the measurement of oxygen tends to be in the mid 20% range. When they measure the oxygen content in an air sample from a big city with few trees and many cars, the oxygen percentage is in the midteens. Oxygen samples from inside buildings are even worse, as low as 10%.*

Even more eye opening is that when scientists took ice samples from three thousand years ago and measured the oxygen content of the air bubbles, they found that it was about 40%. As we continue to cut down trees and pollute the air, we are slowly depriving ourselves of the most vital "nutrient" on the planet.

how to breathe

An important rule for optimal breathing is that breathing should be through the nose, not the mouth. An old saying states that the mouth is for eating and the nose for breathing. That is good advice.

The nose has many functions during breathing. As the air enters the nose, it is filtered by hair that can trap dust and other particles that otherwise might end up in the lungs. The nose contains mucus membranes that will further filter tiny particles, moisten the air if it is dry, and warm the air so it is more usable by the lungs. As the air continues its journey, glands help to fight off germs and bacteria. The ancient yogis believed that prana is absorbed in the nose and not as much when breathing in through the mouth.

We have forgotten how to breathe. With a little practice, we can easily relearn this crucial function.

the three-part breath

The instructor in a yoga class will often talk about the three-part breath. The first part is when you fill the bottom of the lungs with air, followed by the middle of the lungs, and finally the top. Some people have a difficult time learning this technique, but the following is an easy way to learn a complete three-part breath. Your body will do it naturally for you.

- In a comfortable position (seated, standing, or lying down), breathe out through your nose completely until you have no more air. You cannot breathe in fully until your lungs are empty.

- Pause for a moment.

- Breathe in slowly. You will notice that your belly expands first, and then you expand a little higher, and finally the chest slightly expands. That is a three-part breath.

- Pause for a moment.

- Repeat.

Focusing on the exhale and completely emptying your lungs will result in a natural three-part breath. Of course, you should make this one continuous breath and not broken up into three parts. It is important not to strain at any time, especially when bringing the breath into the chest. The flow of breath should be slow, steady, and rhythmical.

breathing for asana

A very important part of stretching is the breathing. Many people tend to hold their breath when stretching. By holding the breath, you increase your risk of injury and won't become very flexible. When breathing slowly and deeply, the nervous system that controls the muscles relaxes. A relaxed mind and relaxed nerves enable optimal stretching without much effort.

There are many different theories about the best way to breathe while doing asana. I will discuss a way that is beneficial to most, but not everybody, and not in every circumstance. You should breathe in a way that feels most natural to you. Remember, the most important part is to breathe. Do not hold your breath. In general:

Inhale as you prepare to stretch

Exhale moving into the stretch

Breathe slowly and deeply while holding the stretch

Exhale coming out of the stretch

Let's see what that looks like while practicing rag doll pose:

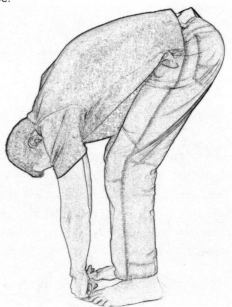

- Stand in a comfortable position, feet hip width apart. **Inhale**.

- **Exhale** and bend forward at the waist. Keep the knees bent to prevent stretching the hamstrings too deeply (these muscles are typically too long). Let the torso and arms hang comfortably with head toward the floor.

- Hold the pose for 1–2 minutes while **breathing slowly and deeply.** You should feel a stretch in your low back. You can stretch a little deeper after each inhale. It should feel comfortable.

- Take one last inhale while in the bent forward position, and **exhale** as you move back to the upright position.

- This general breathing pattern can be applied to most poses.

breathing for optimal health

"When the breath is unsteady, all is unsteady; when the breath is still; all is still. Control the breath carefully. Inhalation gives strength and a controlled body; retention gives steadiness of mind and longevity; exhalation purifies body and spirit." —Goraksasathakam

Many intentional breathing practices can help us to achieve health and well-being. The one I am going to teach you is easy to do (with a little practice) and will bring excellent results. I call this my "health breath." This breath is suitable to practice while sitting, standing, or even lying in bed.

- Find a comfortable position that does not compress your diaphragm.

- Exhale until you have no more breath.

- **On the inhale,** breathe through the nose to a count of 4. The lungs will fill with oxygen that will be distributed by the bloodstream.

- **Hold the breath for a count of 4.** The mind will start to be still. It is said that God resides in the space between the breaths.

- **Exhale to a count of 8.** The lungs will start to eliminate the toxins that have built up.

If you are too challenged breathing in for 4, holding for 4, and exhaling for 8, any of the following ratios will work:

4-4-8

3-3-6

2-2-4

Having the exhale twice as long as the inhale increases the benefits of a breathing practice. You will lower your heart rate, normalize your blood pressure, and your muscles will relax. The longer exhale will also eliminate more toxins in the lungs, such as carbon dioxide, and make it easier to take a full three-part belly breath with no effort.

According to the American Institute of Stress:
Abdominal breathing for 20 to 30 minutes each day will reduce anxiety and reduce stress.
Deep breathing increases the supply of oxygen to your brain and stimulates the parasympathetic nervous system, which promotes a state of calmness. Breathing techniques help you feel connected to your body—it brings your awareness away from the worries in your head and quiets your mind.

—American Institute of Stress http://www.stress.org/take-a-deep-breath/

safety of breathing practices

These breathing exercises I have given you are generally considered safe; however, observe the following precautions:

- If you suffer from asthma, emphysema, dizziness, heart conditions, shortness of breath, or are pregnant consult your physician before attempting these exercises.
- It is important not to strain at any time, especially when bringing the breath into the chest. The flow of breath should be slow, steady, and rhythmical.
- Do not practice breathing techniques after eating a heavy meal.
- Start with five minutes of practice and work up slowly to twenty to thirty minutes.
- Focus on the breath by watching your breath go in and out. Do not let your thoughts wander. This will take some practice to perfect, but it is worth the effort.

starting a breathing practice

If you think you don't have time for a breathing practice, please reconsider. It is the most valuable practice for mental and physical well-being. In my experience, it is more valuable than asana practice.

Here are some ideas on how to be mindful throughout the day and increase the quality of your breaths:

- Set a time each day that you will devote to your breathing practice. An easy way to accomplish that is to practice for ten minutes while you are lying in bed before you go to sleep and ten minutes while you are lying in bed before you get up.
- Breathe while you are doing other activities. Standing in line at the grocery store, waiting for a red light, walking the dog, and riding the bus, for example, are great times to be mindful and breathe.
- After awhile, you will notice that you are breathing more fully throughout the day. Remember that this is a practice. Keep practicing! You will soon start to feel the benefits, which will make you want to practice even more.

In the next chapter you will learn about the many benefits of meditation. Meditation can heal the mind, body, and spirit. You will begin to understand why the ancient yogis considered this the ultimate practice.

Key Points

- **Pranayama** is a Sanskrit word that translates to "control of the breath." I like to think of it as intentional breathing.

- **An important rule for optimal breathing** is that breathing should be through the nose, not the mouth.

  - **Taking a full breath calms the nervous system and reduces stress and anxiety.**

  - **Taking a full breath helps alleviate muscular pain.**

  - **Taking a full breath increases the vital energy in the body.**

  - **Make your exhale twice as long as your inhale.**

  - **Exhaling fully removes more toxins from the body.**

  - **Taking a full breath during asana practice lets your muscles stretch deeper.**

- **A very important part of stretching is the breathing.**

- **If you are thinking you don't have time** for a breathing practice, please reconsider. It is the most valuable practice for mental and physical well-being, even more valuable than asana practice.

CHAPTER 12

meditation—training the mind to heal

"The secret of health for both mind and body is not to mourn for the past, not to worry about the future, or not to anticipate troubles, but to live in the present moment wisely and earnestly."

—Buddha

The ancient spiritual practice of yoga was focused on ways to control the mind and its thoughts as a path to finding union with the Divine. The word yoga means "union." The first seven limbs of yoga were practices to achieve the eighth limb, which is union with God. The ancient yogis also discovered that meditation has many physical and emotional benefits as well.

Meditation is truly a miracle medicine that can heal the mind, body, and spirit. Scientists have now confirmed through numerous studies that meditation is the most effective way to cultivate the power of thought. It's a safe and simple way to enhance our physical, emotional, and mental well-being. Focusing our attention will alter brain wave patterns that will help us reduce stress, alleviate many types of pain, and allow us to thrive in all areas of our lives.

fun fact: The ancient yogis believed that pranayama was more beneficial than asana and that meditation was more beneficial than pranayama.

what is meditation?

The word meditation originates from the Latin word "mederi," which means to heal. This healing covers all facets of dis-ease including physical, mental, emotional and spiritual disease. Some use meditation for spiritual purposes and some for the physical benefits.

Meditation is often thought to be involved with religion, but it is better to view it as a way to know yourself and who you really are. It is the science of training the mind and your thoughts. Many different forms of meditation have been developed to help one achieve this goal. One type of meditation is simply called mindfulness, that is, being present in the moment and not living in the past or future.

Most of our thoughts come from our subconscious mind. The subconscious runs much like an automatic program on a computer. It retrieves the experiences and memories from your entire life. These experiences and memories determine how you think and act. How you think and act determines what you will experience in your life. Therefore, much of your life is spent responding to situations in the exact same way every time, as the subconscious determines how you react to life's situations. Until you start looking at the thoughts and behaviors the subconscious program is running, your life will not change much and you will keep getting the same results in your life. If you want your life to be different in some way you must become aware of your subconscious thoughts.

Meditation can be thought of as a technique to still the mind by focusing within. The mind then becomes clear and relaxed, and thoughts slow down and eventually cease. This will change the brain wave patterns and produce a more desirable state of consciousness. These brain wave patterns also help reduce stress and pain levels in the body.

how does meditation work?

The feelings you feel and the thoughts you think produce different brain wave frequencies that activate different parts of the brain. When you learn to produce different brain wave patterns, you learn to control your state of mind. Cultivating this skill will lead to improved focus, health, and well-being.

Meditation lowers our brainwave patterns from the normal waking consciousness of beta brain waves to the slower states of alpha, theta, and delta brain waves. Each of these brain wave frequencies have many powerful health and well-being benefits.

Let's look at five categories of brain wave patterns:

Gamma (30-100Hz)
This is the state of increased learning and focus often accompanied by sudden insights. When in these frequencies, the brain easily retains information. You feel as if you are in the "zone."

Beta (12-30Hz)
This is the state you experience in the normal waking day, the state of the thinking mind. Beta waves are useful for analyzing, planning, and assessing. Brain waves that slip into high beta, above 20Hz, are associated with stress and anxiety. Your body reacts by releasing the stress hormone cortisol. Increased levels of cortisol can compromise your immune system and promote premature aging. Many people spend a good part of their day in high beta.

Alpha (8Hz-12Hz)
This is the state of slipping down out of the thinking mind, a state associated with awareness, calmness, and relaxation. The brain can produce these frequencies after a walk by the ocean, listening to relaxing music, or participating in a good yoga class.

Theta (4Hz-8Hz)

This is the state between light sleep and waking consciousness. When awake, this frequency is the state where meditation begins. In this state, you can solve complicated problems quickly. Meditators experience inspiration, a sense of wholeness, spiritual connection, and a greater state of awareness.

Delta (1Hz-4Hz)

This is the state of deep, dreamless sleep. Physical healing can occur in this state. Trained meditators have learned how to stay awake while producing these frequencies. Profound spiritual experiences may also occur while in this state.

The purpose, then, of meditation is to get beyond the analytical mind and produce beneficial brain waves that lead to a more enriched life. Listed below is a summary of some of the many benefits of meditation.

benefits of meditation

If you already have a regular meditation practice, you are aware of the many benefits you are receiving. These benefits are often divided into three categories—physical, mental, and spiritual.

Some of the physical benefits include:

• Normalized blood pressure

• Tension-related pain mitigated

• Improvement in immune system

• Slower breathing and heart rates

• Increased energy levels

• Reduced cortisol levels (the stress hormone)

• Ability to sleep better

• Lower risk of heart attack and stroke

Some of the mental benefits include:

• Less stress

• Less anxiety

• Less anger

• More happiness

• More self-esteem

• More mental focus and problem solving

Some of the spiritual benefits include:

• Increased sense of peace

• Increased sense of oneness

• Opened heart

• Increased connection with the inner self

• Increased intuition

In addition to the above benefits, meditation has been shown to naturally release beneficial neurotransmitters that have a profound effect on all facets of our being. The ancient yogis did not have the scientific knowledge about what was happening to them; they had the direct experience. Science tells us that the experiences of the yogis was due to the release of these neurotransmitters during meditation as their brain waves slowly lowered from beta to delta.

Some of these neurotransmitters include serotonin, GABA, dopamine, growth hormone, endorphins, and oxytocin. Let's look at some of their benefits.

Serotonin is a calming hormone. Low levels of this neurotransmitter are a factor in headaches, fatigue, sleeplessness, and anxiety.

GABA is also a calming hormone. People with addictions have one thing in common, and that is a lack of GABA. Research has shown that GABA levels start to rise after only thirty to sixty minutes of meditation.

Dopamine is the happy hormone. It helps to maintain focus and experience pleasure. It helps with sleep and mood.

Growth Hormone is the antiaging hormone. It helps with repair of the body. Lack of this hormone results in fatigue, weak muscles, and weak bones.

Endorphins are the feel-good hormones. Healthy levels of endorphins will help to reduce pain in the body and give a feeling of well-being.

Oxytocin is the pleasure hormone. It produces feelings of contentment and reduces anxiety.

You can begin to see why the ancient yogis called meditation the key to health and well-being.

meditation and pain relief

The benefits of meditation for pain relief are many. Chronic pain affects a staggering one hundred million Americans each year. Many of these people have been suffering with their pain for many years.

I have noticed that my clients have often tried many different approaches to help themselves with their pain. They take up an exercise program, change their diets, and start taking nutritional supplements. These can often bring some relief, but it has been my experience that diets, supplements, and exercise can only take you to a certain stage. Few of my clients have ever told me that they have tried meditation for pain relief.

Numerous medical schools like Harvard, Yale, and UCLA have conducted studies that prove a consistent meditation practice provides significant benefits to those who suffer from chronic pain, stress, and anxiety. Many of these studies can be found in well-respected publications such as The Journal of Pain, The Journal of Neuroscience, and The Journal of the American Medical Association. Lowering brain wave frequencies through meditation can bring dramatic and long-lasting relief from pain, stress, and anxiety, but this will require consistent practice.

Neuroscientists believe that stress reduction is a major component of meditation's beneficial effect on our health. From a muscular viewpoint, emotional stress, which causes a "fight or flight" condition in the body by releasing adrenaline into the system, will make the muscles in the body tighter and more painful. Many of the common diseases in America, such as hypertension and cardiac issues, have stress as a major component. Studies have also shown that people diagnosed with fibromyalgia (widespread pain in the body) have improved by practicing meditation. A person can achieve lower stress levels in as little as four to six weeks of a regular meditation practice.

fun fact: One minute of anger weakens your immune system for four to five hours.

fun fact: One minute of laughter boosts the immune system for over twenty-four hours.

how to meditate

There are numerous forms of meditation practice. Some have a religious focus and some have a secular focus. There is no right or wrong way to meditate. You can meditate while standing, sitting, walking, or lying down. All forms of meditation focus on going within and withdrawing from the external world of thoughts and activities.

Following are two simple and effective meditations. Both will help bring your brain waves down from beta to alpha to theta, and will help release beneficial neurotransmitters that will improve your overall health and well-being.

Choose the one that resonates with you.

meditation on the breath

- Sit comfortably in a chair in Seated Supported Mountain Pose (see chapter 13). This is an easy and comfortable way to sit.
- Gently close your eyes.
- Bring your attention to the breath. Do not try to control it. Simply observe the breath moving in and out of the lungs and nostrils.
- Undoubtedly the mind will wander and begin thinking other thoughts. When this happens, gently bring your attention back to the breath.
- Start by practicing 5–10 minutes a day. You will soon find that you can focus more easily and feel more relaxed.

meditation on a mantra

- Sit comfortably in a chair in Seated Supported Mountain Pose (see chapter 13).

- Gently close your eyes.

- Choose a mantra—a word or phrase you wish to focus on. Simple words or phrases like "peace," "relax," or the Sanskrit word "OM" are best.

- Silently repeat the word over and over. When your mind wanders, gently bring your attention back to your mantra.

- Start by practicing 5–10 minutes a day. You will soon find that you can focus more easily and feel more relaxed.

That is it. You are meditating! You may also find more ways to meditate on the Internet and/or from a skilled yoga teacher. Find the form that resonates with you. Anyone can meditate and enjoy all the benefits that it bestows.

tips for meditating

People have practiced meditation for thousands of years. Following are some tips that will help you learn this beneficial practice:

- Find a quiet place.

- Consistency is the key. Like learning any new skill, practicing every day will bring the quickest results. If every day is not possible, try to meditate at least four or five times a week.

- Start by meditating for five minutes a day and work up to twenty minutes.

- Shorter meditations done every day are more effective than longer meditations done sporadically. Remember, we are training the mind.

- You do not need to meditate at the same time every day, but doing so will help to establish a positive habit. First thing in the morning or just before bed works for many people.

asana, pranayama, and meditation practice

Following is an example of a thirty-minute yoga practice that combines asana, pranayama, and meditation. Combining these three practices brings the peak benefits for body, mind, and spirit, a complete recipe for superior health.

Asana: 20 minutes (5 minutes of warmups and 15 minutes of stretching and strengthening). Choose from the warmups and poses I have given you in previous chapters. There is no need to perform the entire sequence.

Pranayama: 5 minutes. Practice the health breath I described in chapter 11. You may also use any other breath system you have been practicing that works for you. You may do this sitting on your mat in a comfortable seated position or in a chair in Seated Supported Mountain Pose. The most important part of the sitting is that it is comfortable. I prefer sitting in a chair.

Meditation: 5 minutes. Practice either of the two meditations described in this chapter or any other form of meditation that resonates with you. You may do this sitting on your mat in a comfortable seated position or in a chair in Seated Supported Mountain Pose. Again, the most important part of the sitting is that it is comfortable.

Practice daily if possible, but at least three to four times a week. Many people have told me that after practicing meditation and pranayama for a few months, they now spend more time with those practices and less on asana. They have discovered what the ancient yogis knew—asana is only the beginning of yoga. The benefits of a complete yoga practice far outweigh the benefits of asana alone.

I hope I have given you enough information and have inspired you so that you will at least try meditating. Meditation is truly life changing. It will help you to have more positive thoughts and feelings, and you will be happier and have less pain in your life. You will start to see patterns where you are stuck and be able to break free and create better outcomes in your daily activities.

In the next chapter we will look at the many ways that yoga can be incorporated into daily life off the mat. These simple practices will help you to have a better quality of life. Yoga off the mat will bring much quicker results.

Key Points

- **Scientists have now confirmed through numerous studies** that meditation is the most effective way to cultivate the power of thought. Focusing our attention will alter brain wave patterns that will help us reduce stress, alleviate many types of pain, and allow us to thrive in all areas of our lives.

- **The ancient yogis believed that pranayama was more beneficial** than asana and that meditation was more beneficial than pranayama.

- **The word meditation originates from the Latin word *mederi*,** which means to heal. This healing covers all facets of dis-ease, including physical, mental, emotional, and spiritual dis-ease.

- **The feelings you feel and the thoughts you think produce** different brain wave frequencies that activate different parts of the brain. When you learn to produce different brain wave patterns, you learn to control your state of mind. Cultivating this skill will lead to improved focus, health, and well-being.

- **Diets, supplements, and exercise can only take you to a certain stage.** Lowering brain wave frequencies through meditation often brings dramatic and long-lasting relief from pain, stress, and anxiety.

- **One can achieve a lower stress level** in as little as four to six weeks of a regular meditation practice.

yoga off the mat

"Even after you have rolled up your mat,
yoga continues"
—Zubin Atre

as we have discussed throughout this book, correcting muscle imbalances while practicing the yoga poses I have described will result in better posture and less pain. However, you will achieve even better results, and more quickly, if you are willing to incorporate some strategic stretching and strengthening into your everyday life. What you do with your body off the mat is sometimes more important as on the mat. It will also behoove you to be mindful of how you are using your body during the day when you are not on the mat. You need to adjust how you use your body during certain activities so that it is biomechanically efficient. Some of the muscle imbalances you have are avoidable by doing your everyday activities smarter. Some of the imbalances are not avoidable, but they are correctable.

common activities that cause muscle imbalances

As discussed often in this book, sitting—in a chair, at a computer, in a car—can be harmful. Bodies were not designed for sitting in a chair, but since we must sit, we should do it the best way possible—the way that will cause the least amount of muscle imbalances and pain.

People generally sit in a chair one of two ways. Many will sit on the edge of the chair and keep the body straight and aligned. That is, of course, the way the body should look when sitting. The problem, as everyone knows, is that sitting upright on the edge of your chair is not sustainable. After much practice, some people can achieve this standard, but most people will not be able to. Telling someone to sit up straight is the right idea, but it is not going to work for most people. When trying to sit straight in a chair, the back muscles are engaged trying to hold the body upright. For short periods of time that is a good strengthening exercise. If, however, you have to sit for two hours, that is way too long to be strengthening a muscle.

The other and most common way that people sit in chairs is by slouching. I call this slouching "slump asana." The truth is, slouching in a chair feels good at first. The reason is that when slouching in a chair, you are gently stretching your low back. That feels good. Keeping your low back in a stretched position for hours, however, does not feel so good. This slouched position also keeps the hip flexors short, juts the head and jaw forward, and rounds the shoulders. We are developing more and more into a head-forward society. The electronic devices we use require us to look down. In addition to slumping, if we are looking at our devices a good part of the day, the head is being trained to be forward. This leads to pain in many areas of the neck and shoulders.

The head was designed to balance on top of the spinal column. The spine should be bearing the weight of the head. When the head is forward, the muscles become engaged in trying to hold the head up. Many people, as they get older, start to bend forward. I often hear people say that is because they are getting older and it happens to most everyone. But most older people are bent forward simply because they practice being bent forward by doing "slump asana." Your muscles will do exactly what you train them to do.

Mechanical engineers have figured out that for each inch the eight-to-twelve-pound head goes forward, the mechanical strain on the neck muscles increases substantially. For example, if the head weighs ten pounds and protrudes forward one inch, the mechanical strain on the muscles and discs in the neck is twenty pounds. At two inches forward the strain is thirty pounds, and at three inches forward, the mechanical strain is forty pounds.

That amount of weight leads to many neuromuscular problems. The muscles of the neck were not designed to hold up the head in a static position for long periods of time. The result, of course, will be neck pain, headaches, upper back pain, and jaw pain. This will also lead to weak muscles in the upper back that sometimes will develop into kyphosis (a rounded back).

how to sit without pain (seated supported mountain pose)

I have come up with a solution that seems to work quite well for most people. The goal is to sit perfectly straight, but with no effort. That requires a lumbar support of some kind. Any lumbar support will offer some help, but I have not found a ready-made lumbar support that is adjustable enough or soft enough to support the body comfortably. Instead, I recommend using an ordinary bed pillow or travel pillow. The pillow you will use for your lumbar support needs to be on the thinner side so you can roll it to different degrees of thickness. Since every chair and body is built differently, each chair requires the pillow to be rolled to a different thickness. Some people have tried rolling up a blanket or towel. This works for a short period, but ultimately the blanket or towel are not soft enough and they start to dig into the back.

Try this for yourself: Sit up straight in a chair.

Roll up the pillow and place it in the lumbar curve in the small of the back, just above the belt line. Many people place it too low and it is then on their sacrum. It needs to be in the lumbar area.

Make it either thicker or thinner until your head comes back over your shoulders and your body is now sitting up perfectly straight without any effort. Notice that when done correctly, you will be sitting on the sitz bones.

Adjust as needed to make the pillow feel comfortable. If it is too thick, it is uncomfortable. If it is too thin, the head is forward of the body.

If using the pillow causes increased pain or a sharp pain, discontinue and see your doctor. It could indicate a disc issue.

I call this position of sitting with a rolled-up pillow, **Seated Supported Mountain Pose.** This pose, when practiced consistently, will eliminate a great deal of pain in the body. In this comfortable, seated position, bring the focus to the breath and gently deepen each inhalation and exhalation, focusing on bringing the breath deeper into the belly. The breathing will calm the nervous system, and the mind will have less distracting thoughts.

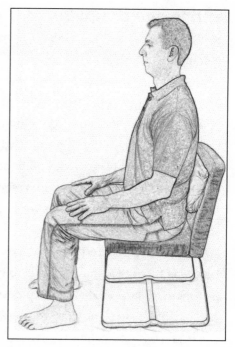

Start practicing Seated Supported Mountain Pose and your pain will lessen, your posture will improve, and you will look years younger.

You can find a free video of how to sit with a rolled-up pillow on my website: www.leealbert. com. I recommend using Seated Supported Mountain Pose when sitting for long periods of time— typically in the car, at the computer, and when meditating.

driving a car

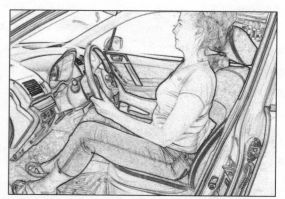

Practice **Seated Supported Mountain Pose** when sitting in a car to take a lot of the strain out of driving. Also pay attention to where your hands are placed on the steering wheel. Most of us were taught to drive at the 10 and 2 position on the wheel. This position, when held for a long period of time, can cause a great deal of pain in the shoulders and neck. Try this for yourself. Imagine you are driving. Now reach out your arms and hold the imaginary steering wheel at 10 and 2. You will likely notice a lot of discomfort in the shoulders and neck. Imagine how it would feel after hours of driving.

To remedy this, hold the steering wheel at 4 and 8 with your elbows by your side. You will notice that the muscular tension is far less. From an ergonomic viewpoint, this is a much better position that will help alleviate neck and shoulder pain. Most states now teach their new drivers to drive at the 4 and 8 position. This helps avoid potential trauma to the face if the air bags deploy.

sitting at a computer

Seated Supported Mountain pose is also recommended when meditating.

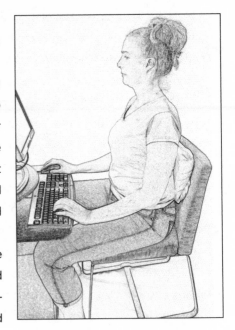

Practice **Seated Supported Mountain Pose** when sitting at your computer. Bring the keyboard and mouse as close to you as you can. Make sure your elbows are by your side. Your monitor should be right in front of you and the screen at eye level so you don't have to look up or down, right or left. Do not rest the wrists or arms on the armrest of the chair. Arms should be bent about 90 degrees. This will also help alleviate neck and shoulder pain.

Laptop computers are not ergonomically friendly. The best way to work with a laptop is to buy a separate keyboard and mouse. Place the laptop on a desk with several books under it so it is eye height. Connect the keyboard and mouse and use it as a desktop computer.

Interesting note: Many of my clients report experiencing a great deal of pain after reading in bed at night. Reading while lying in bed may cause neck and shoulder imbalances that lead to various types of pain. I would not recommend reading in bed unless you are sitting up straight.

off-the-mat exercises that correct common muscle imbalances

The following exercises can be incorporated into your everyday life. The body is like a car. As long as it is being used, it requires maintenance. The exercises below will give some ideas of what to do based on where your pain or discomfort is located. These are easy to practice in everyday life. Many can be done while watching TV, standing in line at the grocery store, or even lying in bed. The most important benefit of these exercises is that they will help keep your body in balance, if you do them consistently.

For Shoulder and Neck Pain

Place the arm on top of the head and let it rest in that position with the head tilted toward the painful side. This position will relieve tension in the shoulders, especially the upper traps and the levator scapula. You may also do this standing or sitting. Hold for at least one minute. Repeat as necessary.

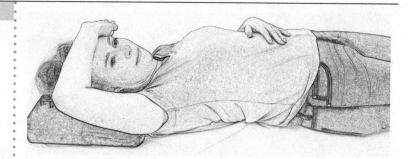

For Shoulder and Neck Pain

Gently squeeze your shoulders up toward the ear. Hold for five seconds. Repeat many times through the day.

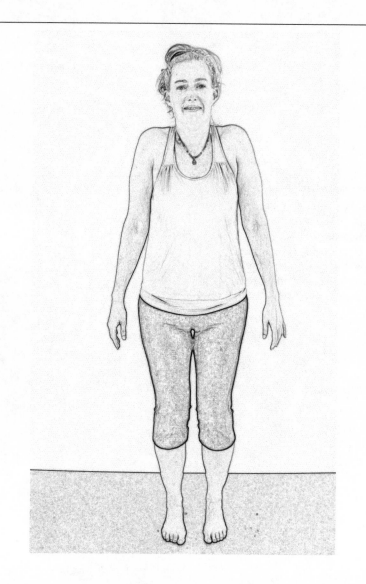

For Wrist and Elbow Pain

Gently twist your palm so your thumb faces down. Hold at least one minute. This will release tension in your lateral elbow and wrist. Repeat as necessary.

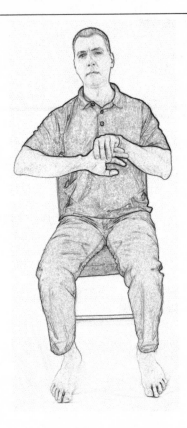

For Upper Back Pain

Hold your hands behind your back. This will release tension between your back and your shoulder blades in the muscles known as the rhomboids. Hold for at least one minute. Repeat as necessary.

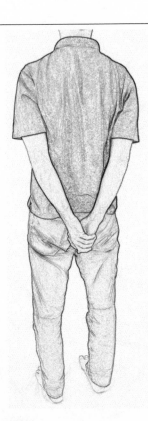

For Low Back Pain

Lie on your back on the floor. Bend at the hip 90 degrees and at the knees 90 degrees. Rest the lower legs on a chair or sofa. Relax in this position for two minutes or longer. This will release tension in the low back. Repeat as necessary.

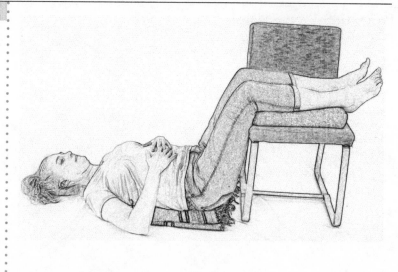

For Neck Pain

Pull your head forward until you feel a slight stretch. Gently push backward into your hands for five seconds. Pull your head forward into a deeper stretch. Repeat as necessary. This will stretch the muscles in the back of your neck. Do not stretch too deeply as this muscle is usually overstretched.

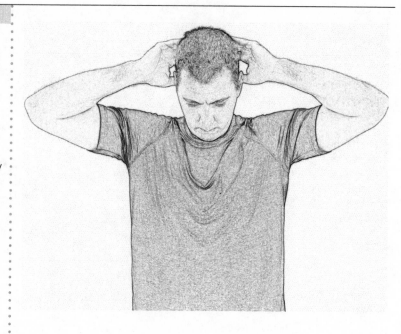

For Neck Pain

Pull head to one side until you feel a slight stretch. Gently push back into your hand for 5 or 6 seconds. Pull head to side into a deeper stretch. Repeat as necessary. Repeat on other side. This will stretch the muscles on the side of your neck.

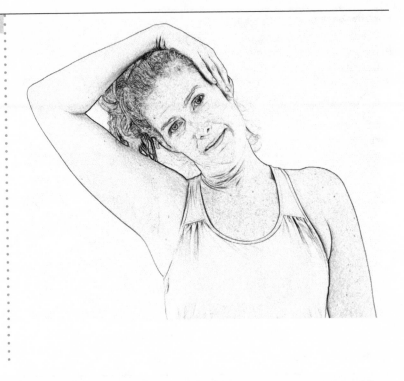

For Neck Pain

Rotate the head to one side until you feel a slight stretch. Gently rotate back into your hand for five or six seconds. Rotate the head to the side into a deeper stretch. Repeat as necessary. Repeat on the other side. This will stretch the muscles on the front of your neck.

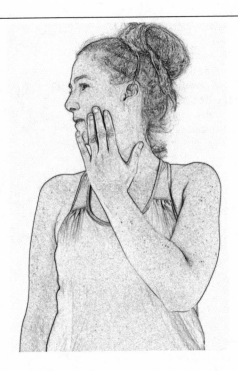

For Knee Pain

Sit with your feet slightly turned in and feet under the chair. This will take strain off the low back and the knees.

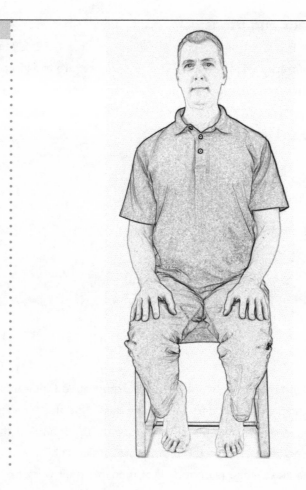

Caution: If any of the above positions or stretches causes pain or discomfort, don't perform them for now. As your body starts to come into balance, these exercises will likely start to feel good.

the daily 5 for better posture and less pain

In my private practice, I consistently recommend four stretches and one strengthening exercise to my clients. Most people will benefit from practicing these exercises. Make them a part of your daily routine, and you will be training your muscles to give you better posture and less pain. They can also help with increased energy and mental clarity.

- Stretch the quads
- Stretch the psoas
- Stretch the hip abductors
- Stretch the chest
- Strengthen the hip extensors

stretch the quads and psoas

Almost everybody has short flexors (predominantly rectus femoris and psoas). This implies that the hip extensors (predominantly hamstrings and glutes) are too long. Short hip flexors and long hip extensors are the cause of many painful conditions. Here is a list of some of the conditions that have short hip flexors as part of the root cause:

- Low back pain
- Sciatica
- Lumbar disc issues
- SI pain
- Gluteal pain
- Knee pain
- Foot pain
- Groin pain
- Neck pain
- Yoga butt

If everyone stretched their hip flexors and strengthened their hip extensors, the issues listed above would be significantly reduced. One of the best antidotes for sitting is to practice stretching the hip flexors and strengthening the hip extensors both on and off the mat as the best antidote for sitting. You sometimes hear the term "yoga butt" talked about in yoga class. If you observe the students in a yoga class, you may notice that many of their buttocks stick out more than usual. They have a pronounced lumbar curve. This means they have an anterior tilt of the pelvis due to excessive hamstring stretching (forward folds). When you are performing forward folds, you are making your hip flexors shorter. Less stretching of the hamstrings and more stretching of the quads and psoas will remedy "yoga butt" and the conditions I have listed above.

Following are some great off-the-mat stretches for the quads and psoas. Remember that if your knees, back, or groin hurt while doing these stretches, then you are stretching too deeply. If your hamstrings cramp, you are also stretching too deeply. Your body is giving you a clear signal that you are stretching too deeply.

Stretch the quads and psoas three to five times a day. Hold for 30–60 seconds.

Quad Stretch

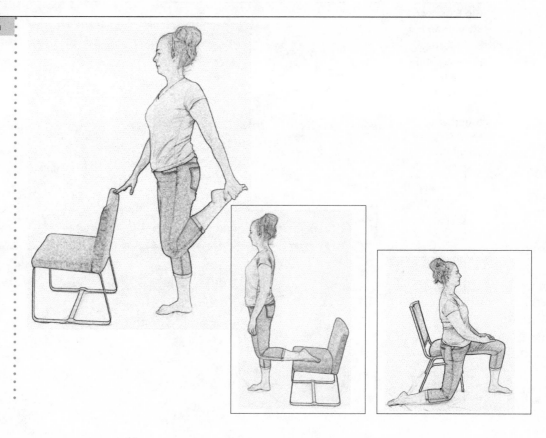

Psoas Stretch

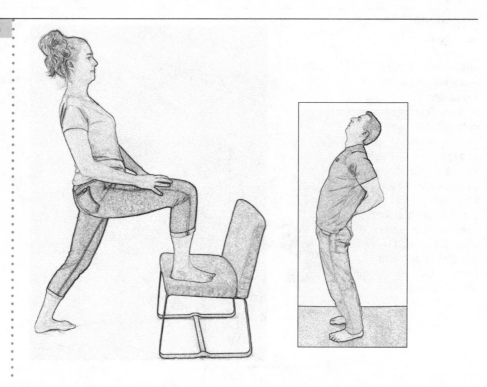

Hip Extensor Strengthening

Practice these exercises three to five times a day. Squeeze gluteal muscles together. Hold 30–60 seconds.

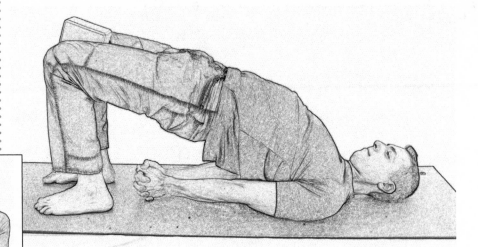

Hip Abductor Stretch

Stretching the hip abductors will help to reduce or eliminate many hip and knee issues. Most of us walk with our feet rotated outward. This puts abnormal strain on the hip and knee joints. The following stretch will help to correct this issue. This exercise also gives you a better chance at keeping your original hips and knees. Practice this stretch three to five times a day and hold for 30–60 seconds.

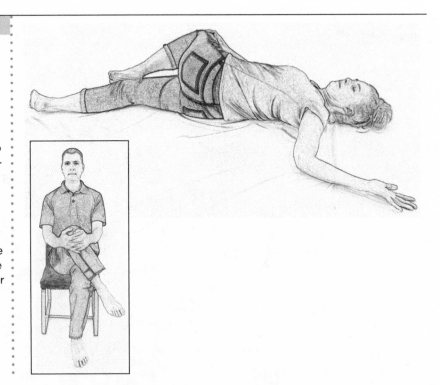

Chest Stretch

We are a forward bent society. This leads to many painful conditions in the upper back, neck, and shoulders. Stretching the chest every day will start to open the chest and bring the head back over the shoulders. This will eliminate or reduce a lot of discomfort in the neck and shoulder area and also train the muscles to help you stand up straight even as you age. Practice this stretch three to five times a day. Hold for 30–60 seconds.

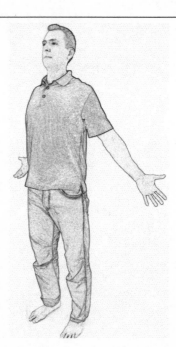

Caution: Never stretch into a painful position. You will achieve better results by being gentle. Choose the version of the exercise that feels better to you. The goal is not to stretch as far as possible but to slightly increase range of motion. These exercises have been proven to be effective when done consistently and gently.

Key Points

- **To achieve even better results and more quickly,** incorporate some strategic stretching and strengthening into your everyday life.

- **I have noticed that three activities** that most people perform on a daily basis cause at least 50% of all the pain I treat—sitting in a chair, sitting in a car, and sitting at a computer.

- **Start practicing Seated Supported Mountain Pose** and your pain should lessen, your posture should improve, and you will look years younger.

- **I find myself consistently recommending four stretches and one strengthening exercise** to my clients. Make these a part of your daily routine, and you will be training your muscles to give you better posture and less pain.
  - Stretch the quads
  - Stretch the psoas
  - Stretch the hip abductors
  - Stretch the chest
  - Strengthen the hip extensors

endnotes

page 16

A great deal of research presents evidence that the root cause of many neuromuscular pain patterns is due to biomechanical malalignments caused by muscle imbalances. Therapists often refer to this as the muscles being locked long or locked short.

> Wolf Schamberger, *The Malalignment Syndrome: Diagnosing and Treating a Common Cause of Acute and Chronic Pelvic, Leg and Back Pain* (Elsevier, 2013).

page 18

Misalignment of the skeletal structure caused by muscle imbalances can cause compressions of the nerves, discs, and other structures in the body. It can also cause the fascia to be twisted and restricted. Fascia is a band of fibrous connective tissue enveloping, separating, or binding together muscles, organs, and other soft structures of the body. These twists, compressions, and tight muscles ultimately lead to less oxygen in the tissues at those areas. The medical term for this is ischemia, which means that the blood getting to the tissues is inadequate. Since blood is the carrier of oxygen, the tissue is not getting enough oxygen. **This lack of oxygen is the source of a lot of pain.**

> "Ischemia Causes Back Pain," Sensei Adam Rostocki, The Back Pain Authority, accessed April 4, 2017, http://www.cure-back-pain.org/ischemia.html.

page 19

An example of this is the person with an anterior pelvic tilt (excessive arch in the low back). As the pelvis tilts forward, the hamstrings are lengthened. Over time, these muscles begin to feel "tight." In most cases, the individual will feel the need to stretch the hamstrings. As the hamstrings are stretched, the GTO (Golgi tendon organ) will inhibit the muscle spindles (autogenic inhibition) and the hamstrings will begin to feel as though they have relaxed. Yet this altered position of the pelvis causes a lengthened resting position of the muscle, and as soon as the GTO is no longer excited, the muscle spindle will begin to signal for the CNS to contract, leading to recurring tightness.

> "Overactive Versus Underactive Muscles: What Does It All Mean," Kyle Stull, NASM.org, accessed April 4, 2017, http://blog.nasm.org/newletter/overactive-versus-underactive-muscles-mean/.

page 34

Mark Singleton has pointed out in his book *Yoga Body: The Origins of Modern Posture Practice* (2010, Oxford University Press) that modern yoga practice is substantially different from the ancient practice and has borrowed many of its ideas from European gymnastics and strength training. There is little evidence to support the theory that the ancient yogis practiced asana for health and fitness.

> Mark Singleton, *Yoga Body: The Origins of Modern Posture Practice* (New York: Oxford University Press, 2010).

page 34

In a rare interview, BKS Iyengar, the ninety-year-old ambassador of yoga to the West, told me that his yoga, as taught to him by his master, was a purely physical exercise and completely un-related to ancient philosophy. He says he invented and refined much of it himself. It wasn't until 1960, while on a visit to London, that English intellectuals introduced Iyengar to the ancient "yoga sutras." Five years later, he combined the yoga poses and the Hindu teachings together in his book *Light on Yoga*, which then sold hundreds of thousands of copies in the United States. And voila— the modern yoga craze was born. But it was basically a new age invention, not an ancient practice.

> "Going to the Mat: Confessions of a Yoga Guinea Pig," Nicholas Rosen, Huffington Post, May 14, 2009, http://www.huffingtonpost.com/nicholas-rosen/going-to-the-mat-confessi_b_186332.html.

page 36

Research has shown that when the muscles are in balance, many painful conditions are eliminated and range of motion increases.

> Wolf Schamberger, *The Malalignment Syndrome: Diagnosing and Treating a Common Cause of Acute and Chronic Pelvic, Leg and Back Pain* (Elsevier, 2013).

page 43

As yoga has become more popular, injury rates have been steadily rising. It is imperative that yoga teachers and yoga students become more aware of the contraindications as it relates to their situation.

> "Insight From Injury," Carol Krucoff, Yoga Journal, August 28, 2007, http://www.yogajournal.com/article/lifestyle/insight-from-injury/.

page 45

Sports MDs have observed that many injuries in yoga are from repetitive strain, pushing too hard to achieve a pose and not listening to the body. They further state that they have seen many hip injuries that lead to osteoarthritis and eventually to hip replacements.

> "Yoga Regimes and Poses Pushed Too Far Can Lead to Hip Injuries, Even Osteoarthritis, Sports MDs Say," Sheryl Ubelacker, The Canadian Press, November 26, 2013, http://life.nationalpost.com/2013/11/26/yoga-regimens-and-poses-pushed-too-far-can-lead-to-hip-injuries-osteoarthritis-sports-mds/?__federated=1.

page 48

Overstretching can lead to pain and inflammation in the soft tissues themselves or in the joints. Symptoms of inflammation include redness, swelling, heat, and pain. An example would be Achilles tendonitis. Some of the latest research has indicated that inflammation is not part of the problem but is actually the body's response to a condition and is part of the healing process. In any case, inflammation is a sign of a problem.

"Inflammation Helps to Heal Wounds—Surprise Discovery," Robert George, Medical News Today, October 6, 2010, http://www.medicalnewstoday.com/articles/203538.php.

page 115

In many studies, slow, deep breathing for as little as ten minutes has been shown to calm the sympathetic nervous system, reduce stress and anxiety, and bring the body back into homeostasis (balance).

"Dr. Herbert Benson's Relaxation Response," Marilyn Mitchell, MD, Psychology Today, March 29, 2013, https://www.psychologytoday.com/blog/heart-and-soul-healing/201303/dr-herbert-benson-s-relaxation-response.

page 118

According to the American Institute of Stress: Abdominal breathing for 20 to 30 minutes each day will reduce anxiety and reduce stress. Deep breathing increases the supply of oxygen to your brain and stimulates the parasympathetic nervous system, which promotes a state of calmness. Breathing techniques help you feel connected to your body—bringing your awareness away from the worries in your head and quieting your mind.

"Take a Deep Breath," Kellie Marksberry, AIS, accessed April 4, 2017, https://www.stress.org/take-a-deep-breath/.

page 121

Meditation is truly a miracle medicine that can heal the mind, body, and spirit. Scientists have now confirmed through numerous studies that meditation is the most effective way to cultivate the power of thought.

"The Science of Meditation," High Existence, accessed April 4, 2017, http://highexistence.com/the-science-of-meditation/.

page 130

Mechanical engineers have figured out that for each inch the eight- to twelve-pound head goes forward, the mechanical strain on the neck muscles increases substantially. For example, if the head weighs ten pounds and protrudes forward one inch, the mechanical strain on the muscles and discs in the neck is twenty pounds. At two inches forward the strain is thirty pounds, and at three inches forward, the mechanical strain is forty pounds.

"Forward Head Posture," Erik Dalton, PhD, Dalton Myoskeletal, November 15, 2010, http://erikdalton.com/blog/forward-head-posture/.

bibliography

Anderson, Dale L., MD, *Muscle Pain Relief in 90 Seconds: The Fold and Hold Method* (New York: John Wiley & Sons, Inc., 1995).

D'Ambrogio, Kerry J. and George B. Roth, *Positional Release Therapy: Assessment & Treatment of Musculoskeletal Dysfunction* (St Louis, Missouri: Mosby, 1997).

Dispenza, Dr. Joe, *Breaking the Habit of Being Yourself: How to Lose Your Mind and Create a New One* (New York: Hay House Inc., 2012).

Dispenza, Dr. Joe, *You Are the Placebo: Making Your Mind Matter* (New York: Hay House Inc., 2014).

Edwards, Michaelle, *YogAlign: Pain Free Yoga from Your Inner Core* (Hanalei, HI: Hihimanu Press, 2011).

Kravitz, Judith, *Breathe Deep Laugh Loudly: The Joy of Transformational Breathing* (Center Sandwich, NY: Ini Free Press, 1999).

Long, Ray, *The Key Muscles of Yoga* (Baldwinsville, NY: Bandha Yoga, 2006).

McAtee, Robert E. and Jeff Charland, *Facilitated Stretching* (Champaign, IL: Human Kinetics, 2007).

Satchidanada, Sri Swami, *The Golden Present: Daily Inspirational Readings* (Buckingham, VA: Integral Yoga Publications, 1987).

Schamberger, Wolf, *The Malalignment Syndrome: Diagnosing and Treating a Common Cause of Acute and Chronic Pelvic, Leg and Back Pain* (Elsevier, 2013).

Scheumann, Donald W., *The Balanced Body: A Guide to Deep Tissue and Neuromuscular Therapy* (Baltimore, MD: Lippincott Williams & Wilkins, 2007).

Singleton, Mark, *Yoga Body: The Origins of Modern Posture Practice* (New York: Oxford University Press, 2010).

thank you

I want to personally thank you for your dedication and commitment to your own individual self-care and for taking your care and compassion out into the world. By sharing the ideas in this book, I hope you will be able to practice yoga more consciously and experience superior benefits.

We are at a time in the world when traditional medical models often have no long-term solutions for what we feel in our bodies. Intuitively, we feel a need for the knowledge that can help us heal our own bodies. We feel a need to learn how to be less stressed without drugs and how to have happiness as we journey through life. I have been helping people for twenty-five years to achieve a pain-free life. It has been my experience that the protocols discussed in this book have helped thousands of individuals to have more ease in their bodies and more calm in their hearts.

We all have a hand in weaving a new future for the world. Together, we are making a difference! I believe we are on this planet to help each other. There can be no greater aspiration than to help your family, friends, and neighbors achieve a more fulfilling life by having less pain and stress, and more peace and happiness. The Dalai Lama said it best: "When we feel love and kindness toward others, it not only makes others feel loved and cared for, but it helps us also to develop inner happiness and peace."

It is my utmost desire that the information contained in this book will be of some value on your journey while you are on this planet. Try what I have suggested and see for yourself that you are capable of helping yourself lead a more empowered and fulfilled life. I wish you much peace, happiness, and, of course, a pain-free life.

acknowledgments

I would like to take this opportunity to gratefully acknowledge the work of some amazing people whose contributions were invaluable.

To my models Andy Steigmeier LMT, CSCS and Laura Jensen for never complaining when we had to shoot the same photo over and over to make me happy.

To my photographer Karla Archambeault who made sure every detail of the photos were correct and kept everyone happy and on track.

To my illustrator Philip Nato who redrew the anatomical drawings without a single complaint until I figured out what I really wanted.

To Marcia Albert, my wife, to Vickie Gillhouse and Josh Warren M.S., my students and friends, who so willingly gave of their time to read the manuscript and were able to figure out what I was really trying to say and then helped me choose just the right words.

I give each of you a very heartfelt thank you for your love, support and expertise. Your contributions have meant everything to me.

—Lee Albert, NMT

about the author

Lee Albert, NMT, creator of Integrated Positional Therapy (IPT), is a nationally recognized yoga instructor and expert in neuromuscular pain relief. For over 25 years, Lee has helped people learn how to live pain-free using IPT's innovative tools and techniques. He treats patients one-on-one at the Kripalu Center for Yoga & Health in Lenox Massachusetts. Lee conducts training seminars in IPT, Pain Free Yoga and consults with businesses on ergonomic training for employees to reduce workplace injuries. Connect with Lee at www.LeeAlbert.com

index

The page numbers for major discussions of a topic are shown in **bold** typeface. Illustrated asanas are shown by page numbers in *italic* typeface. Modified poses (e.g. modified Pigeon Pose) will be found under Pigeon Pose.